ARE YOU AT RISK?

- Have other members of your family suffered from osteoporosis?
- Are you underweight?
- Do you smoke?
- Do you consume heavy amounts of alcohol?
- Is your calcium intake low?
- Do you take medications that could cause bone loss?
- Do you live a sedentary lifestyle?
- Have you broken a bone after the age of forty?

THE OSTEOPOROSIS CURE

Reverse The Crippling Effects
With New Treatments

HARRIS McILWAIN, M.D.
and DEBRA FULGHUM BRUCE

AVON BOOKS ⬥ NEW YORK

The ideas, procedures, and suggestions in this book are intended to supplement, not replace, the medical advice of a trained medical professional. All matters regarding your health require medical supervision. Consult your physician before adopting the suggestions in this book, as well as about any condition that may require diagnosis or medical attention. The authors and publisher disclaim any liability arising directly or indirectly from the use of this book.

AVON BOOKS
A division of
The Hearst Corporation
1350 Avenue of the Americas
New York, New York 10019

Copyright © 1998 by Harris H. McIlwain, M.D. and Debra Fulghum Bruce
Published by arrangement with the authors
Visit our website at **http://www.AvonBooks.com**
Library of Congress Catalog Card Number: 97-94411
ISBN: 0-380-79336-9

First Avon Books Printing: May 1998

AVON TRADEMARK REG. U.S. PAT. OFF. AND IN OTHER COUNTRIES, MARCA REGISTRADA, HECHO EN U.S.A.

Printed in the U.S.A.

OPM   10   9   8   7

To our families: Linda, Laura, Hugh, Kim,
Michael, Ginah, Lisa, and Danny;
Bob, Rob, Claire, Brittnye, and Ashley

Acknowledgments

Ashley Bruce
Brittnye Bruce
Hugh Cruse, M.S.P.H.
Kim McIlwain
Laura-McIlwain Cruse
Mike McIlwain
Rick Ruge, Supervisor, Media Services,
    University Community Hospital

Contents

ONE

Osteoporosis: When Thin Is *Not* Beautiful

If you are young or middle-aged, it is difficult to believe that osteoporosis could affect you. If you are an older but active adult, breaking a bone or losing height as a result of this disease may be hard to comprehend. After all, your bones probably seem sturdy enough, and you are still active and able to do what you want in life. But osteoporosis is a quiet and accomplished thief. There are no visible signs until fractures occur. Your body can harbor it quietly for years, then suddenly normal stress on bones from sitting, standing, coughing, or hugging a loved one can cause fractures that lead to chronic pain and immobility. With repeated fractures, this debilitating bone condition gradually leads to more painful fractures, disfigurement, and immobility.

Many consider osteoporosis to be a normal part of aging; this disease is *not* normal, yet at some point, it will crush the active lives of *more than half of all women over age forty-five.* No one wants to be haunted by her own skeleton, and she needn't be because osteoporosis *is* both preventable and treatable.

So much myth and lack of information surround this bone disease that most patients are shocked when they receive the diagnosis of osteoporosis and want to know exactly why their bodies have failed them. Many are surprised to find out that this disease did not happen overnight but usually took many years to manifest. One patient, seventy-two-year-old Marian, had trouble believing that osteoporosis caused her fractured ankle, then later a fracture in her spine. She asked if we could operate to "remove the osteoporosis." There is *no* surgery to remove or treat osteoporosis. Yet using the treatment plan in this book, you can take measures to halt, reverse, and stop the fractures from this disease!

Simply stated, *osteoporosis is thinning of the bones— a decrease in the density of bones.* This is one instance in which the word *thin* is not coveted. Over time, as bones become weaker, they become easier to fracture or break. For millions of older adults with the disease (about 75 percent are women), such daily activities as walking, bending, or even opening a window may be stressful enough to cause a broken bone. These fractures commonly occur in the back, the hip, the shoulder, and the wrist. In fact, with this disease a seemingly minor injury that in normal circumstances would go unnoticed can result in a fracture with severe pain, limitation and expense.

A CONCERN FOR ALL PEOPLE

Years ago, osteoporosis was considered a normal result of aging like wrinkles or gray hair. It has only been in recent years that researchers have defined osteoporosis as a specific disease that we can prevent. Until the past decade, this disease used to be an older woman's concern, particularly women over age sixty. Newer research repeatedly warns that osteoporosis is a concern for *all people*, no matter what their age or gender. In fact, 25 percent of osteoporosis and fractures happen in men, including hip and spine fractures. It appears that such risk factors as cigarette smoking, excessive alcohol, lung disease, exercise habits, and medications contribute to bone loss in men. Likewise, men who have relatives with this disease are found to be at greater risk of bone loss.

Today's figures are startling. Osteoporosis currently affects more than thirty million people in our country. While women have a one-in-eight chance of developing breast cancer in their lifetime, by age sixty-five they have a *one-in-two chance of fracturing a bone due to osteoporosis*. The tragic result is that more than *half* of all postmenopausal women will experience fractures that could be avoided if they adopted the preventive and treatment plans.

BUILDING PEAK BONE MASS

The most critical time to build bone is during the teenage years. Generally, our bone mass peaks between ages twenty-five and thirty. However, some women reach this peak before age twenty. Then the tide turns. At some point, usually around thirty-five or later, women begin to lose bone, sometimes at a rate of 1 percent per year. This loss jumps up to about 4 percent per year during the five to ten years after menopause (usually age forty-five to fifty-five). For those who did not drink their milk during childhood and adolescence, or for those with several risk factors, this loss could be critical.

While previous recommendations were to guard against osteoporosis *after* menopause, newer research shows that bone loss *can and must* be treated much earlier—at the ages of thirty, forty, and fifty—*long before fractures and deformity occur*. With today's medical breakthroughs and the greater understanding of osteoporosis, you now can avoid bone fracture, dowager's hump, and even loss of height!

THE BONE-BUILDING CYCLE

Before you see how to diagnose, prevent, and treat this debilitating disease, it is important to understand the bone-building cycle. Bone is not a lifeless structure. Rather, it is complex, living tissue. As if on schedule, our bodies constantly break down old bone and rebuild new bone. This process is called "remodeling." In children, more bone is built than removed, so during this life stage, bones become larger and stronger. In fact, the skeleton reaches about 95 percent of its peak amount of bone by age twenty.

After age thirty to thirty-five, the amount of bone our bodies break down begins to catch up with the amount of bone our bodies are building. Sometime during this period, the bone removed equals the bone built. Then usually after age forty, the mass of bone removed can surpass the bone which is built. It is at this time that osteoporosis disrupts the natural bone-building cycle, resulting in a decrease in the amount of bone in our bodies.

At menopause, hormonal changes disrupt this bone-building cycle again. Specifically, the natural decline in estrogen at menopause speeds up the breakdown of bone. During the five to ten years after menopause, there is a greatly accelerated loss of bone mass in women. Many women have lost a startling *25 percent of their bone density within the first five years after menopause.*

This may be difficult to comprehend for active women in midlife when good health is taken for granted. At this life stage it is estimated that *fewer than 10 percent of those who have osteoporosis actually know they have it and are treated.* Many don't arrive at this knowledge until they fracture a bone. Seventy-five percent of women with osteoporosis have not been diagnosed or treated.

If the decline in bone continues over a period of ten to twenty years, bones become thinner, weaker, and easier to break or fracture. Though painful, the break will heal. Yet as long as the bones are thin and weak, they are increasingly susceptible to fractures and the resulting immobility or even death.

If such fractures only affected fingers or toes, it would be inconvenient but not terribly limiting. However, osteoporosis commonly attacks with painful vengeance. It leaves fractures in those bones that allow us to be active and enjoy life: the bones of the spine, the wrist, the shoulder, and the hip. These fractures cause severe limitation and prevent victims from doing their daily activities. Fractures, especially when they affect the spine, can also cause deformities. None of this has to happen to you as you can treat osteoporosis, build stronger bones, and end fractures forever.

NOT FOR WOMEN ONLY

Although osteoporosis and fractures are more common in women, men are also at risk. In fact, osteoporotic fractures in men are a serious, neglected public health problem as more than *1.5 million* men in this country already have this disease, and *3.5 million more* are at high risk of getting it. Men start with stronger, heavier bones, yet by age sixty-five, many men have a similar rate of bone loss as women.

The main risk factor for men is *age*. While men do not have a sudden decline in bone mass at middle age the way postmenopausal women do, their more subtle losses add up. In fact, the longer a man lives, the greater his chances are of suffering a fracture due to osteoporosis. After age eighty, *one in four men* will suffer a broken hip, and *one man in seven* will have a spinal fracture sometime in their lives. Don't forget, while a small amount of bone loss or thinning can occur naturally with aging, in osteoporosis a larger loss of bone happens to make bones fragile enough to break.

There are many conditions that increase a man's

chances of getting osteoporosis before sixty-five. Lung disease such as emphysema and chronic bronchitis, low testosterone hormone levels, cigarette smoking, heavy alcohol, prostate cancer and its treatment, and certain medications such as cortisone drugs can cause men to lose bone at an earlier age. Like estrogen in women, testosterone in men plays an important role in bone maintenance. In older men, the level of testosterone commonly drops.

COMMON CAUSE OF FRACTURES

With the revolutionary breakthroughs in our nation's health care, we all are living longer. However, as the population ages, we can expect the alarming incidence of osteoporosis to soar over the next twenty years.

Let me give you a clear-cut example of what is in store. In the late 1990s, more than *fifty million* women will turn fifty (four thousand every day!), making this the largest group of women ever to hit menopause. Most of these women will live at least one third of their lives *after* menopause. Soon *one person out of six* will be over age sixty-five (see table 1.1). We are an aging nation and can expect to see the number of hip and other fractures increase unless we take action.

Osteoporosis is the most common cause of fractures, causing 1.5 to 2 million fractures each year, resulting in more than sixty thousand persons admitted to nursing homes and fifty thousand deaths. This long-term care adds to increased disability with escalating hospitalization and rehabilitation demands and a total annual cost for hip fractures alone exceeding twelve to fifteen billion dollars.

Within the next ten years, this cost is expected to skyrocket to twice this amount ... unless we take action to prevent this disease immediately. The number of fractures will also escalate over the next few years as the projected population over age sixty-five increases. One study recently predicted *4.5 million* annual hip fractures worldwide by the year 2050.

In the midst of staggering statistics, there is some positive information. Using the newer methods of detecting osteoporosis, along with the latest medical treatments described in this book, fractures can be prevented and the risk of hip fracture can now be *reduced by up to 50 percent* even for women who already have osteoporosis. Now, there is no need to suffer from a fracture—if everyone takes personal responsibility for the health of her bones.

HIP FRACTURE

"Aren't I a bit too young for a bone density test? Hip fractures only happen in the elderly," a forty-year-old woman said as I scheduled her for her first bone density test. Untrue! While general bone loss among women begins in the perimenopausal period (the years prior to menopause), bone loss from the hip begins even earlier. In fact, this woman's bone density score was lower than other women her age, and she was also found to be at higher risk for future fractures.

Table 1.1
Projected Percentage of the U.S. Population
Age 65 and Over
Headed for Osteoporosis

% over 65	12.8%	12.9%	13.4%	16.3%	20.1%	20.7%
Year	2000	2005	2010	2020	2030	2040

Think about how a hip fracture would affect you. Hip fractures can be serious injuries, often a turning point beyond which independent living is no longer possible. Perhaps you have a friend or family member who was active and living alone—until she fell and broke her hip. For those who suffer hip fracture, recovery can be difficult as they face hospitalization, surgery, and months of painful, exhausting, and expensive therapy.

Sadly, statistics show that in the first year following a broken hip from osteoporosis, an average of *one in five* of these patients will die, a statistic that increases with age. By age seventy-five to eighty, a fall and broken hip can result in up to *50 percent* chance of death within a year. Comprehensive studies reveal that while more than *one hundred thousand men* fracture hips annually, of these, *more than thirty-three thousand or one third die*. Now that we can treat osteoporosis, build bone mass, and prevent hip fractures, this statistic could decrease dramatically.

Although there are several different areas in the hip that may break, most are referred to as a "hip fracture." The fracture almost always requires surgery, since without surgery it would take six weeks or more of bedrest for fractures to heal. With surgery, the patient can usually be up and walking within a few days. The operation to correct these fractures is expensive, around thirty thousand to forty thousand dollars or more. Along with this cost comes the higher risk of other serious medical problems such as blood clots, heart attack, pneumonia, and stroke. Even worse, many of these victims immediately lose their independence and up to one third never regain it.

I could tell you about the radically changed lives of hundreds of patients who have suffered with hip fractures, many of whom have moved to nursing homes or become totally dependent on family members and friends. One in particular is Dotty, a vivacious sixty-five-year-old woman who had a hip fracture just one month after retiring from teaching fifth grade in the public school system.

Dotty had been active her entire life and was planning to travel across the United States with her husband of forty-five years. They had even purchased a recreation vehicle to use for their yearlong trip. Instead, a short fall off a step at her daughter's home resulted in a severely fractured hip and robbed Dotty of this dream. She spent weeks in a rehabilitation center. The financial cost of hospitalization, surgery, recovery, and rehabilitation was phenomenal, but the personal cost of suffering to Dotty and her family could never be totaled.

Measuring the personal costs of hip fractures is difficult. For example, *half* of those who break a hip never walk as well or even walk alone again. About *one third* become totally dependent on others for their daily activities. And how do we measure the cost of lost independence?

Have you seen an older person who was living independently in her home or apartment—until she fell and broke a hip? This person goes from enjoying independence and good quality of life to losing her home, her independence, and her circle of friends because she can no longer care for herself. This tragedy not only affects the patient but extends to family, friends, and health care professionals as they must now provide full-time caregiving.

You may be reading these statistics and wondering, "Is the outlook really so gloomy? What if we could detect and treat this disease *before* these fractures occur? Can you imagine the savings in suffering and expense that might happen?"

Osteoporosis does not have to be gloomy! As you will learn in Chapter 3, detecting osteoporosis is *now* possible and easy with a simple, painless bone density test. Steps for prevention and treatment are also painless and easy, as outlined in Chapters 4 and 5. New medications, can build bone mass and help keep you fracture-free.

SPINE FRACTURES

By age seventy-five, more than 50 *percent* of women have had a fracture in their spine, with an estimated half million vertebral fractures occurring annually. The most common deformity from osteoporosis, called the dowager's hump, happens in the upper part of the back from these fractures.

Osteoporosis is the most common cause of loss

of height as we age (see figure 1.1). In the dowager's hump, each fractured vertebra becomes shorter, usually by one-fourth inch, causing the spine to bend forward. The person will appear stooped over, which makes the abdomen prominent. One of my patients said that she went from a height of five feet four inches as a young woman to four feet eleven inches at age seventy-five.

As bones become thinner and weaker, the weight of the body while standing or walking may be enough to cause a fracture. Bending and lifting can greatly stress the spine, often putting pressure equivalent to several times the weight of the body on the back. This pressure leads to fractures in weakened bones.

After age forty-five, men and women may lose a small percentage of their height annually. However, doctors actually consider osteoporosis in any person who loses height. When osteoporosis affects the spine, fractures can happen in one of the vertebral bones. If each fracture in the spine can cause about one-quarter inch loss of height, after many fractures there may be a loss of several inches in total height. Treatments described in Chapter 5 have been shown to help *delay* the shortening and deformity of the spine that causes the stooped posture.

When osteoporosis is present and weakens the bones, it is a wonder that sufferers do not experience more fractures in the spine. Science tells us that lifting an *eighty-six-pound* object from the floor can place *seven hundred pounds* or more of force on the back. One fifty-seven-year-old woman said that she had her first spinal fracture, along with weeks of excruciating pain, after merely opening

Table 1.2
Reasons Why We Shrink Other
Than Osteoporosis

- Poor posture
- Disk deterioration
- Muscle weakness

her bedroom window. She was completely bedridden for a week from her pain.

Fractures in the spine cause back pain that can be severe, making it difficult to stand, walk, sit, or lift. In some cases, the pain can be so excruciating as to make the smallest movement difficult and almost any position uncomfortable. This can cause loss of independence as we can no longer care for ourselves and our families. How can we take care of a home when there is severe pain with almost any movement, along with an increased risk of more fractures?

Once a spinal fracture occurs, the pain may worsen when you try to walk, bend, or lift. This pain commonly prevents sleep at night. You may feel penetrating pain when you cough or sneeze. (Pain from a spinal fracture does not usually travel down the legs, so if you have this feeling, let your doctor know.)

Sometimes you may fracture more than one bone in the spine, resulting in pain that lasts for weeks. If pain is severe for longer than a few days, check with your doctor—there may be an additional problem in the spine. If you notice a change in your bladder or bowel habits, such as loss of control, then call your doctor to be sure no other serious problems are present.

WRIST AND SHOULDER FRACTURES

The wrist and the shoulder are also common places for osteoporosis to attack; in fact, it causes *more than two hundred thousand wrist fractures* annually. Fractures in these bones usually happen after a fall. It is easy to overlook the fact that a disease is involved in the fracture. Osteoporosis may be found when your doctor examines an X ray. As discussed in Chapter 3, the simple bone density test can be administered to let your doctor know if further treatment is needed to prevent the next fracture.

Fractures of the wrist or shoulder may need an operation to repair, but most do not require a hospital stay and can be treated on an outpatient basis by an orthopedic surgeon. After the bones heal, you may need to see a physical therapist or do exercises at home to be sure you do not lose use of these areas for daily activity.

PELVIS FRACTURES

These fractures usually happen after a fall, with an injury to the bones of the pelvis, causing great pain in the pelvis, lower abdomen, and groin areas. This often requires days or weeks in bed or in the hospital. After a pelvic fracture, walking is

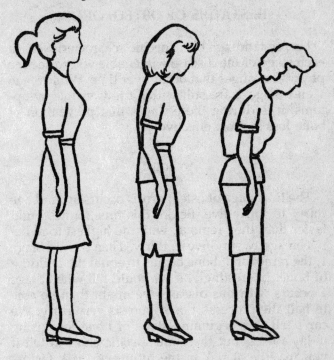

Figure 1.1 – A young woman, middle-aged woman, and elderly woman, showing normal spine, then bending of spine and loss of height due to osteoporosis.

very painful. After a few days to a week, most patients can stand. Then, after a few more days, they can begin to walk again. If osteoporosis is found, steps must be taken to prevent more fractures.

THE STAGES OF OSTEOPOROSIS

Understanding the specific characteristics in each stage of the disease will enable you to see the physical changes that occur over time. While Stage 1 and Stage 2 are still without any visible symptoms, it is during these stages that prevention of bone loss is most effective.

STAGE 1

The first stage of osteoporosis occurs around age thirty to thirty-five. Before this time, bones build faster than they remove, with the highest total between age twenty-five to thirty. Then during Stage 1, the removal of bone begins to equal the building of bone. Interestingly, if we could tell when Stage 1 occurs with this disease, we might then be able to halt the process of osteoporosis very early. We can't tell this beginning stage of bone loss using today's tests, but there are specific clues to tell if you may be at risk in the future (see risk factors on page 34). Once these clues are identified, you can make lifestyle changes to halt or slow the progression of the disease, even before symptoms are evident.

STAGE 2

In the second stage of osteoporosis, usually after age thirty-five to forty-five, overall bone mass decreases. Over a period of several years, the breakdown of bone continues at a much faster pace than the body builds bone. It is during this second stage that osteoporosis first becomes detectable with bone density tests. The bones may still be strong enough to prevent unusual fractures, and there are still no overt signs or symptoms to alert you to the possibility of the disease.

Simple and safe tests, such as DXA (dual-energy X-ray absorptiometry), are available to discover osteoporosis in Stage 2. As discussed in Chapter 3, these tests are virtually lifesaving measures as they can detect the disease years before a fracture occurs. If it is detected at this early point, specific steps, including the use of bone-building medications, can be taken to slow or stop the disease. However, if Stage 2 continues undetected, the bones gradually grow thinner over the years until a break occurs. Because everyone with this disease is different, bone loss occurs at varying rates. This makes it even more important to find out your own bone density.

STAGE 3

Stage 3 of osteoporosis usually happens after ages forty-five to fifty-five. Rate of bone loss varies from individual to individual, and some people even younger than forty-five can reach this stage. One thirty-eight-year-old mother of two small children was recently diagnosed with Stage 3 after suffering from three broken ribs after a fall. You may lose bone faster or slower than others, depending on these factors:

• a fracture after age forty
• estrogen replacement therapy after menopause

- activity level
- calcium intake
- family history
- certain medications
- lifestyle habits such as smoking or drinking alcohol
- onset of menopause

During Stage 3, bones eventually become so thin that they break from stress which normally strong bones could withstand. Fractures that seem out of proportion to the injury are often due to Stage 3 osteoporosis. For example, a minor trip over a garden hose results in a fracture of the ankle in three places. Or lifting a bag of groceries out of the car causes a fracture in the spine. One of my patients broke two ribs when her small grandson hugged her! We diagnose most cases of osteoporosis during Stage 3 after this first fracture has occurred.

STAGE 4

In Stage 4 of osteoporosis, the fractures continue, the pain increases, and disability sets in. Deformities in the spine and other areas may become much more obvious. There may be more difficulty getting around and doing daily activities because of the pain and stiffness. The good news is that this stage is becoming less common as treatment is available to prevent future fractures. Even at this stage, it is never too late to begin treatment.

NO MORE FRACTURES

If you or those you care about wait for signs or feelings of osteoporosis, then you will wait for

Table 1.3
The Stages of Osteoporosis

	STAGE 1	STAGE 2	STAGE 3	STAGE 4
Age	30 to 35	35+	45+	55+
Symptoms	None	None	Fractures	Fractures
Signs	None	None	Fractures	Pain and deformity
Detection	None	Bone density tests	Bone density tests	Bone density tests

painful, debilitating fractures. There are no other signs. By the time a fracture occurs and you are alerted to the disease, osteoporosis has been present for many years, slowly leaving your bones brittle.

It does not have to happen this way. If you learn nothing else from this book, I want you to remember this: *Fractures do NOT have to happen!* Interestingly, some new studies have found that if we could stop bone loss after the age of fifty-five (or after menopause), the number of fractures in women would *decrease* by almost 40 percent!

The decades before a fracture occurs are the critical years when you can treat the disease and keep bones strong. Having received this advice, you must realize that it is *never* too late to try to prevent fractures, but *the most important fracture to prevent is the first one.*

TWO

Evaluating
Your Risk

Until recent years, I rarely diagnosed patients with osteoporosis until they came to me in most unfortunate ways—with painful, fractured bones. Terri, a secretary for a law firm, suffered her first fracture at the age of fifty-three. This once active mother of three had worked full-time in a sedentary job for more than a decade. She had no regular exercise program, lived on coffee and cigarettes to keep her weight down, and rarely drank milk or ate calcium-rich foods. Although Terri was in great pain with a fractured ankle, it may have saved her life.

Using the DXA bone scan, as discussed in Chapter 3, this woman was found to have a bone density of only *60 percent* of normal—she had lost 40 percent of her bone! After a thorough discussion, including review of her family history, this woman was shocked to hear that she had almost every risk factor for the disease—many of which she could control. Let's look at Terri's list of risk factors:

- Caucasian female
- small bone structure
- low dietary calcium
- both mother and grandmother had osteoporosis and fractures
- an early menopause at thirty-five (hysterectomy)
- no estrogen replacement therapy (ERT)
- a cigarette smoker (two packs a day)
- sedentary job and no regular exercise program

Luckily, Terri recovered from her ankle fracture in a few weeks. She then made it her goal to take control of her health and to halt osteoporosis. Reviewing her risk factors, obviously she could not change her age, sex, or family history. Yet she could quit smoking, add calcium supplementation to her diet, walk several miles a day, and take one of the new medications to help build bone strength. For Terri, growing older without the fear of another fracture was enough reward to make all these dramatic lifestyle changes.

Osteoporosis usually does not choose its victims at random. Instead, there are specific environmental and genetic risk factors that influence osteoporosis. Although these risk factors do not actually cause the disease, they can be excellent indicators to alert you to the underlying problem.

As you read about the following specific risk factors, you will realize as Terri did that there are some we cannot change, including our family history, race, having had a fracture after age forty, sex, and age. In contrast, there are crucial risk factors that *can and must be changed*, including lack of regular exercise, cigarette smoking, body weight (underweight), heavy alcohol use, certain medications, low calcium intake, and, at times, even excessive exercise.

While many factors influence osteoporosis and can serve as clues, sometimes people have *none* of the risk factors and still have the disease. I have a few patients who have none or only one risk factor for osteoporosis and still have low bone density. On the other hand, some of my patients have several risk factors yet show no measurable loss of bone.

RISK FACTORS FOR FRACTURES THAT *CANNOT* BE CHANGED

We acknowledge that certain risk factors cannot be changed and must be accepted. Look at the following, and see how many describe you or your family.

- **A family tendency**. "Like mother, like daughter" may especially be true in osteoporosis. If one of your natural or biological family members has had a broken hip, frequent fractures, loss of height, or stooped posture from osteoporosis, you may be at increased risk for the disease. We do not know the exact reasons, but it is likely that an inherited genetic code in some way raises the likelihood of this disease in certain families.

  Some researchers have found that our inherited genetic programs may be major factors in deciding how strong our bones become before age thirty. Besides affecting how strong our bones are at their peak, our genetic inheritance may also affect how quickly we lose bone after age thirty to thirty-five.

- **Race**. Race also is part of our inherited genetic makeup. Research has shown that having a Caucasian background places you at the highest risk of osteoporosis and fractures, especially for women. Having Hispanic or Asian genetic background may place you at an intermediate risk, while African-American genetic background typically has the lowest risk for osteoporosis and fractures.

  As a group, African-Americans show a higher peak bone density between thirty to forty, and a slower rate of bone loss after forty. In fact, the overall risk of hip fracture in African-American women is about *one half* that of Caucasian women. Some recent research suggests that this statistic may be changing, with many postmenopausal African-American women losing bone as fast as Caucasian women.

- **Bone fracture after age forty.** Although the reasons are not known, researchers have shown that if you have a fracture after age forty, then your risk of having another fracture is about twice as high as normal.

- **Sex and age**. After age thirty to thirty-five, our bodies produce bone at about the same rate as we break it down. Then, in the mid-thirties or later, bone removal begins. This can happen in both sexes, but is more common at an earlier age in women than men. At the usual time of menopause, age forty-five to fifty-five, osteoporosis and fractures greatly increase in women as estrogen production by the ovaries decreases and the rate of bone loss accelerates (see The Stages of

Table 2.1
Risk Factors You Can't Change

(Age)

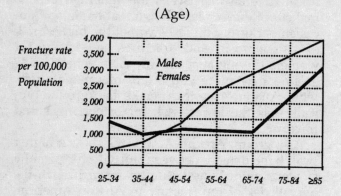

Osteoporosis on page 16). The use of estrogen treatment can greatly improve this risk factor, prevent bone loss, and change the shape of the line on the chart for women (Table 2.1).

As men age and as life spans increase, so does the risk of fractures. This can be caused by low levels of testosterone associated with aging, chronic diseases, prolonged exposure to cortisone drugs or other medications, and lifestyle patterns such as smoking, drinking, lack of exercise, and a diet low in calcium. If a man lives to age seventy-five to eighty, the risk of having a hip fracture may be as high as *25 percent*.

One patient, Thomas, age eighty-two, had been healthy and active most of his life when he was diagnosed with prostate cancer. After undergoing radiation and medical therapy for several months, he tripped on the stairs at home and fractured his hip. In the hospital, a bone density test revealed that Thomas had Stage 3 osteoporosis.

If this fall and hip fracture had occurred ten years ago, the prognosis would have been bleak. But Thomas started on Fosamax (alendronate), a new medication that actually increases bone mass, along with a diet high in calcium. Although he is unable to do a lot of weight-bearing exercises, crucial for keeping bones strong, he still lives a normal, active life with his family and friends, doing the very things he enjoys. In fact, his latest bone density test revealed an increase in bone mass by 5 percent, giving him much hope for a strong, fracture-free future.

RISK FACTORS FOR FRACTURES
THAT *CAN* BE CHANGED

Changing those risk factors over which you have control is one important key to stopping osteoporosis. Read the following, and see if these can be changed in your life.

- **Having regular bone density tests**. The strongest risk factor for fractures is a low *bone density test*. This test can show low bone density and osteoporosis, which means the bones are thinner than normal and cannot stand the same amount of stress and injury as they could in earlier years. A bone density test would explain why a sixty-year-old patient tripped over her granddaughter's stuffed animal during a visit and suffered from fractures of her foot in several places. It would explain why a person loses several inches in height. And it would explain why a seventy-two-year-old man broke his wrist while swinging a golf club in a tournament.

I have many patients, mostly women in their fifties, sixties, and seventies but some even younger, who have broken ribs during a coughing spell—the result of osteoporosis. What is compelling is that the fractures are usually dramatically out of proportion to the injuries. This is most likely because the bones were not as strong as normal, which allowed more serious fractures to occur with less force or stress.

Researchers have found an even stronger correlation between low bone density and fractures than the greatly publicized connection between high blood cholesterol and heart attack or the connection between hypertension and stroke. Who does not accept the value of knowing whether your blood cholesterol or blood pressure is high? Likewise, your bone density score is just as important to your health in preventing future fractures.

Should you take the time and trouble to have a bone density test? If you are a postmenopausal woman, one quick and easy way to tell is the SCORE Test. This is a simple test of six questions selected by researchers. You simply add up your score and you can tell if it would be worthwhile to have a bone density test. If your score is six or higher, then research shows that there is a good chance of osteoporosis and you should check it out with a bone density test.

TABLE 2.2
SCORE TEST

Take the following quiz to assess your risk for osteoporosis.

1. What is your current age? _____ years
   Take this number, multiply by three and enter in this space
                                                    _____
                                                    Start

2. What is your race or ethnic group?
   (Check one)
   ❏ African-American (Enter 0)
   ❏ Caucasian ❏ Hispanic (Enter 5)
   ❏ Asian ❏ Native American (Enter 5)
   ❏ Other (Enter 5)   _____

3. Have you ever been treated for or told you have rheumatoid arthritis?
   ❏ Yes   ❏ No
   If yes, enter four. If no, enter zero.   _____

4. Since the age of 45, have you experienced a fracture (broken bone) at any of the following sites?
   •Hip ❏ Yes ❏ No If yes, enter four   _____
   •Rib ❏ Yes ❏ No If yes, enter four   _____
   •Wrist ❏ Yes ❏ No If yes, enter four   _____

5. Do you currently take or have you ever taken estrogen? (Examples include Premarin, Estrace, Estraderm, and Estratab) If **no**, enter one.   _____
   Yes _____   No _____

Add score from questions one to five.   ____

        Subtotal

6. What is your current weight?
   ____ pounds   ____

Take your weight and subtract from the **subtotal** to
receive your score.   ____

        Score

**If your final score is six or greater, you should be eval-
uated further for osteoporosis. Talk to your doctor.**

If a bone density test shows osteoporosis, your
risk for bone fractures is increased. If you increase your bone density, you can lower your
risk for fractures. Just as treatment is now available for control of hypertension and high blood
cholesterol, treatment is also available to control
osteoporosis and fractures.

• **Lack of regular exercise**. Lack of exercise has
been known for years to increase osteoporosis
and the risk of fractures. This has been found
even in young patients who must stay in bed for
a long time. Without activity, bones become thinner and weaker. It can take patients months to
regain bone strength after prolonged bed rest.
   Even a cast on the lower part of the arm, when
used to treat a wrist fracture, can reduce bone
strength. Researchers have found that patients
who wore a cast on their wrist for three weeks
lost about 6 percent of the bone in that area.

Healthy, young astronauts must deal with lack of weight-bearing exercise on space flights. Although scientists have tried to prevent the loss of bone caused by weightlessness, it is common to see a 1 percent bone loss per month of space time. Remember, this is in healthy, young astronauts!

We spend time on each visit to be sure every patient—no matter what their age—is doing their exercises. They become stronger and their bones become stronger.

- **Smoking cigarettes**. Most people realize the connection between cigarette smoking and lung cancer or other respiratory diseases. But did you realize that cigarette smoking *doubles* your risk of osteoporosis? This is a key risk factor you can control. Research has shown that osteoporosis starts earlier and increases at a faster pace in smokers. While we do not know the exact reasons, experts think some of the many chemicals and substances contained in the smoke may cause this bone loss. The good news is that when you stop smoking, you can lower your risk of osteoporosis by *one half*.

- **Being underweight**. Being underweight for your height increases the chances of osteoporosis and fractures, while being overweight actually lowers the osteoporosis risk! It is possible that having more fat tissue causes more effect of estrogen on the bones to slow osteoporosis. Lean women have the greatest risk of hip fractures. While they typically have low bone mass, they also have low levels of estrogen and little fat to cushion their falls. It is likely that having more fat tissue results in either more production of estrogen by the larger number of fat cells or more

Table 2.3				
1983 Metropolitan Height and Weight Table				
MEN				
HEIGHT		**SMALL**	**MEDIUM**	**LARGE**
FEET	**INCHES**	**FRAME**	**FRAME**	**FRAME**
5	2	128–134	131–141	138–150
5	3	130–136	133–143	140–153
5	4	132–138	135–145	142–156
5	5	134–140	137–148	144–160
5	6	136–142	139–151	146–164
5	7	138–145	142–154	149–168
5	8	140–148	145–157	152–172
5	9	142–151	148–160	155–176
5	10	144–154	151–163	158–180
5	11	146–157	154–166	161–184
6	0	149–160	157–170	164–188
6	1	152–164	160–174	168–192
6	2	155–168	164–178	172–197
6	3	158–172	167–182	176–202
6	4	162–176	171–187	181–207

effect of estrogen on the bones to slow osteoporosis.

Use the Metropolitan Height and Weight tables to assess your weight, then discuss this with your physician if there is a problem.

- **Heavy alcohol consumption**. Excessive alcohol intake can increase the chance of osteoporosis and resulting fractures. This may be because many heavy drinkers do not eat nutritious foods and are malnourished. Interestingly, the evidence so

Table 2.3 continued			
WOMEN			
HEIGHT **FEET INCHES**	**SMALL FRAME**	**MEDIUM FRAME**	**LARGE FRAME**
4 10	102–111	109–121	118–131
4 11	103–113	111–123	120–134
5 0	104–115	113–126	122–137
5 1	106–118	115–129	125–140
5 2	108–121	118–132	128–143
5 3	111–124	121–135	131–147
5 4	114–127	124–138	134–151
5 5	117–130	127–141	137–155
5 6	120–133	130–144	140–159
5 7	123–136	133–147	143–163
5 8	126–139	136–150	146–167
5 9	129–142	139–153	149–170
5 10	132–145	142–156	152–173
5 11	135–148	145–159	155–176
6 0	138–151	148–162	158–179

Weights at ages 25–59 based on lowest mortality. Weight in pounds according to frame (in indoor clothing weighing 3 lbs. for women, 5 lbs. for men, shoes with 1" heels).

The tables are reprinted courtesy of Metropolitan Life Insurance Company, Statistical Bulletin.

far shows that a moderate amount of alcohol—the equivalent of a one-ounce drink, i.e., one ounce of distilled eighty-proof liquor; twelve ounces of beer, or a half bottle of wine or less daily—does *not* increase the risk of osteoporosis.

Some revealing studies show that this modest amount of alcohol may actually help increase the bone density. Too much alcohol can increase osteoporosis, but the exact amount that constitutes "too much" is not known. Some researchers speculate that more than three drinks a day (or more than twelve drinks a week) can lower bone density and contribute to osteoporosis.

- **Medications**. Certain medications may set you up to lose even more bone mass. In fact, corticosteroid drugs can be a major cause of osteoporosis. The most common medications in this group are cortisone derivatives such as prednisone that are often prescribed for such diseases as acute bronchitis, allergic diseases, asthma, chronic obstructive pulmonary disease (COPD), eye diseases, rheumatoid arthritis, and ulcerative colitis, among others. The problem with these medications is that the longer these are taken and the higher the dose, the more likely bone thinning becomes. When corticosteroid drugs are used for longer than one year, the risk of fractures greatly increases. It is important to note that a short course of treatment, such as a few days or a few weeks, is usually not a major risk factor.

Over time, some of the particular medical problems requiring these medications may also bring a greater risk for osteoporosis. For example, rheumatoid arthritis greatly increases your risk for osteoporosis. If a cortisone drug is added, as is commonly necessary in severe cases, the risk may go up unless very low doses are used.

Local injections of a cortisone drug, such as those used for bursitis or tendinitis, do *not* increase the risk of osteoporosis. Likewise, steroid inhalers used for nasal and lung diseases do not usually increase this risk, if kept to a standard dosage.

Other medications that are known to affect bone loss include some drugs prescribed for epilepsy and seizures, thyroid hormones, and certain medications used for treating endometriosis, prostate cancer, or with some fertility treatments. Large amounts of antacids containing aluminum, some cholesterol-lowering drugs, and heparin can also cause bone loss over a period of time.

If you are taking any of these medications, talk with your doctor to see if they can affect osteoporosis. Also, consider a bone density test to measure your bone strength. There are ways to prevent bone loss from medications such as prednisone.

- **Low calcium intake**. It makes sense that if you give your body less calcium than it needs, it will build less bone. While sufficient calcium intake is important for all ages, it is especially important for adolescents since this is the crucial time to build up bones. The chart on page 127 gives the recommended daily amounts of calcium needed to maintain strong bones.

- **Excessive exercise**. Some athletes are at a greater risk for osteoporosis, including those in their late teens and twenties. Women who exercise vigorously in the course of demanding physical training often use strict diet and weight control, which can produce lower levels of estrogen. Their menstrual periods may become irregular or stop altogether (amenorrhea). Almost every sport is affected but especially gymnasts, long-

---

Table 2.4
Check Your Risk Factors for Osteoporosis and Fractures

RISK FACTORS YOU CAN'T CONTROL	RISK FACTORS YOU CAN CONTROL
• Genetic predisposition	• Having regular bone density tests
• Race	• Lack of regular exercise
• Bone fracture after age forty	• Smoking cigarettes
• Sex and age	• Being underweight
	• Heavy alcohol consumption
	• Medications
	• Low calcium intake
	• Exessive exercise in athletes

---

distance runners, soccer players, and other athletes who exercise strenuously for long periods.

Researchers find that 25 to 50 percent of female athletes' menstrual periods have stopped, usually when their body fat drops below 18 percent. Estrogen levels drop and osteoporosis can follow, with fractures which limit their performance.

- **Hip fractures**. Because of the importance of hip fracture in cost, in loss of independence, and in the higher risk of death over a year, researchers have identified specific risk factors to help find those persons at very high risk for hip fracture. By being aware of this higher propensity for a broken hip, you can make necessary changes for prevention and treatment.
- **Injuries and falls**. If osteoporosis is present, then

problems that make falls more likely can increase the risk of hip fractures. Leg weakness, unsteadiness, dizziness, medications that cause light-headedness and alcohol use may all contribute to further falls and hip fracture.

Tripping on objects in the home or workplace greatly raises the risk of hip fracture. Telephone cords, slippery rugs, and darkened rooms from low lighting, especially at night, can add to the chances of falling. See page 81 for more suggestions on fall prevention.

- **Past fractures along with low bone density**. Some researchers have found that if you have had any fracture after age forty and you have a lowered bone density your risk of *hip* fracture may increase by four or five times. These combinations of risk factors are important because they routinely occur and may show us that more careful prevention measures for some persons are warranted.

- **Diminished vision**. Some researchers have found that people who have decreased vision have a higher risk of hip fracture, especially when combined with lower bone density. This seems understandable since the change in vision could certainly make falls happen easier.

Think about an older friend or relative who may have impaired vision. You can get a feeling for her situation if you wear a pair of clear glasses with petroleum jelly rubbed on the lenses. Try this for a few minutes, then try to walk down a set of stairs with these special glasses on. You will see what millions of elderly adults deal with! Add to this experiment a dark-

Table 2.5
Check Your Risk for Hip Fractures

____ Injuries and falls
____ Any past fractures along with low bone
      density
____ Diminished vision
____ Falls to the side directly on the hip

ened room, and the dangers become very apparent.

- **Falls directly on the hip**. Some experts have found that when patients fall and suffer a fracture of a hip, they often fall directly to the side, with the weight on the hip. This has led researchers to devise a prevention program in which hip pads are used that can be beneficial in helping to prevent hip fractures in those who fall. It is best to try and prevent falls altogether since it is difficult to predict which way we will fall.

MAKE POSITIVE CHOICES

No matter how quickly you begin making lifestyle changes to reduce your risk factors for osteoporosis, it is important to know there is no "quick fix" for bone loss. Nevertheless, the positive choices you make today will affect your present as well as future health, if you take control of those risk factors you can change. You can stop this disease. Understanding the disease and how it manifests itself in the bone is vital. However, it is also important to understand the current methods of diagnosis, weigh the advantages of the latest medications to build bone, and begin a lifelong program to improve your bone strength and quality of life.

THREE

Assessing Your Bone Health

In many cases, we *can* take control of our health. Early detection, prevention, and treatment of diseases can make a major difference in later years. For example, avoiding cigarettes prevents most types of lung cancer, as well as chronic bronchitis, emphysema, and other debilitating respiratory diseases. Eating a low-fat diet helps to prevent heart attack and certain cancers. Mammograms can detect early breast cancer, and the prostate specific antigen (PSA) blood test detects prostate cancer at early stages when treatment is most effective.

As in all chronic diseases, early diagnosis and treatment are important in osteoporosis. And it is much easier and cheaper to prevent fractures than to try to regain use after a bone has broken.

Knowledge is power, especially with osteoporosis. Once you have a bone density test, you will know exactly how strong your bones really are—before it is too late. Using this lifesaving information, you can start a prevention or treatment program without the fear of broken bones, immobility, disfigurement, or loss of independence as you age.

Although there is much enthusiasm about the newer bone density tests, it is important to note that this screening is *not* necessary for every woman or man. Key factors such as sex, age, lifestyle habits, and family history should all be taken into consideration before you agree to this test.

After considering her risk factors, Caroline, a forty-seven-year-old health professional, felt that a bone density test was warranted, especially since her grandmother had recently suffered a broken hip and was in a nursing home. Working in the health-care field, Caroline was acutely aware of the increased risk of fractures when other family members are affected. While this woman had not yet reached menopause, she did have a sedentary lifestyle and did not take calcium supplements.

Caroline's DXA bone density test showed osteoporosis and a higher risk of fractures in the future *if* she did not take precautions. She immediately began treatment, including calcium and vitamin D supplements, a daily exercise program of walking and strength training, and medications to build bone strength. Two years later, Caroline has put a halt to bone loss and her latest bone scan already shows improvement in bone strength.

Sixty-year-old Babs is another example of someone who found out she had osteoporosis before having a fracture. This was especially lucky in her case, considering her bone density test showed a significant reduction of *more than 40 percent loss of bone*.

Realizing that she was in Stage 2 of osteoporosis

and at higher risk for a broken hip, Babs immediately began a program that included calcium and vitamin D supplements, exercises to increase bone strength, and medication to help build bone. She knew that if she could increase her bone density, her risk of fracture would lessen. As with Caroline's situation, this treatment program enabled Babs to increase her bone density, as measured by the DXA bone test (see page 45), and reduce her risk of future fractures.

For active women like Caroline and Babs who are considering estrogen replacement treatment (ERT), or men and women who have more than two or three risk factors for the disease, a bone density test is in order. If you have had a broken bone, but your doctor did not mention osteoporosis, a bone density test may bring this diagnosis to light. Then you can begin treatment to lower the risk of future fractures and immobility. Or if you have relatives with osteoporosis yet have no other risk factors, having the bone density test may put your mind at ease about this disease.

Bone density tests may offer more thorough explanations about the devastation of osteoporosis. Using these tests, researchers have found that after a hip fracture, most patients lose even more bone and muscle, perhaps because of the forced loss of activity. Interestingly, one year after a hip fracture, some patients were found to have a *5 to 7 percent* loss of bone density. And the body's overall amount of muscle after one year was found to be reduced by *5 to 9 percent*.

This loss of bone and muscle, along with the sudden loss of strength, may help explain why older patients experience serious problems after a hip fracture. This might also help explain why so many never become independent or walk as well again.

UNDERSTANDING BONE DENSITY TESTS

Bone density tests evaluate the strength of the bones in your body by measuring a small part of one or a few bones. These assessed bones represent the rest of the bones in the skeleton. The areas that are most commonly measured are the hip, the lumbar spine (in the lower back), or the forearm (the lower part of the arm just above the wrist). These test results show how your bone density compares to a normal young adult, as well as to other people your age.

There is more than one way to measure bone strength. Many available tests are quick, easy, and do not cause any discomfort. There is a cost for the test, but the information you gain will be invaluable and could save your life. Some states now require insurance companies to cover these tests if you are at a higher risk. Most health insurers will pay for this test if you have one or more risk factors such as:

- a fracture
- if you are postmenopausal
- if you are not taking estrogen at menopause
- if you are taking medications that can cause bone thinning

Nevertheless, these tests are not as accessible as needed. For example, there are not nearly enough machines on the market to test the millions of men and women at risk. Especially in a rapidly aging society, this limitation represents just one of many reasons why *fewer than 10 percent* of those who have this disease are being treated.

You may wonder if people at risk are really interested in finding out their bone density measurement. Recently a trial program was advertised in Florida, making bone density testing available to women at risk for a very low cost. The test was also convenient (in neighborhood pharmacies). Included in the advertisement was a special toll-free number.

Within a few days, thousands of callers responded. Many of these women were found to have reduced bone density, putting them at risk for osteoporosis and fractures. These women were referred to their physicians for further testing and treatment evaluation. Lifesaving screening programs similar to this are now operating in many cities across the United States.

DECODING THE TESTS

Before you have your bone density test, it is important to understand what the resulting score means. This score will immediately let you know if your bone density is at the point that places you at higher risk for injury and disfigurement. If your score is low, you and your doctor can decide what the best treatment program will be. This treatment may include adding calcium and vitamin D to your diet, starting a regular exercise program, and using medications to build bone. Treatment has been shown to effectively increase bone density, and it is well established that if you increase your bone density, you also lower your risk of fracture. You can prevent fractures!

If you are among those fortunate enough to have a normal score, this means that you are *not* at a higher risk of fracture. Accordingly, you and your doctor can map out the best prevention program, including eliminating all risk factors over which you have control while maintaining a healthy diet and lifestyle to keep bones strong. You can prevent osteoporosis!

WHAT'S NORMAL, WHAT'S NOT

Osteoporosis experts consider normal bone density to be that of a normal, young adult. In the DXA test, this is called a normal "T-score" and has no unusual risk for fractures. Your test result will give this T-score along with the following key values:

1. Your actual result in the DXA test (expressed as grams per square centimeters).
2. Your T-score or Young Adult score (a value for bone mass compared to your approximate expected highest bone mass before menopause). A T-score *of −1.0 or higher* is in the normal range. A score *between −1.0 and −2.0* means that your bone density is borderline for osteoporosis (osteopenia). A T-score of *−2.0 or lower* qualifies as osteoporosis.
3. Your Z-score (which is not used to diagnose

Figure 3.1
T-SCORE

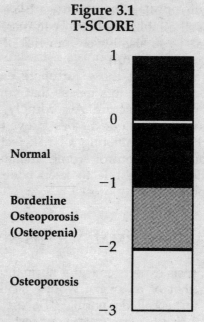

Your T-SCORE shows whether your bone density is normal, borderline osteoporosis (osteopenia) or osteoporosis.

osteoporosis but to give you a comparison to others your age and sex).

Understanding this T-score is quite simple. For example, if you are a fifty-five-year-old woman with a T-score of −2.0, this means that your bone mass measurement is 2 standard deviations (SD) below that of a young adult and your risk of fracture is higher than normal. For every SD below the young adult normal, the amount of bone in the body decreases by about 10 to 15 percent.

Osteoporosis is diagnosed by many researchers and the National Osteoporosis Foundation when the result of your T-score bone density test is −2.0 *or lower*. The World Health Organization calls it osteoporosis when the result is −2.5 *or lower*.

DXA (DUAL-ENERGY X-RAY ABSORPTIOMETRY)

DXA (or DEXA) is the most popular bone density test used today. It is performed when you first realize that you have more than two or three risk factors, or when you have a fracture and osteoporosis is suspected. DXA uses a very small amount of X ray to measure bone mass at clinically relevant sites on the body, usually the hip or lumbar spine. Then this measurement is used to estimate the amount of bone that is present in the rest of the body. The DXA test is quick, taking only a few minutes to complete. You'll be asked to lie down on a table or sit in a chair, but you won't have to undress. No pain or needles are involved.

While ordinary X rays cannot pick up changes in bone density until losses exceed *25 to 40 percent*, DXA is accurate, dependable, and can be used to diagnose osteoporosis very early before fractures occur. It can also determine whether the bone strength has improved with treatment. The DXA scanning time can take as little as five minutes, and the cost ranges from fifty to two hundred dollars for the measurement of one area, such as the hip, spine, or wrist. When osteoporosis is being treated, the test may be repeated in about one year. This gives the treatment time to show an increase in bone strength.

While the test does involve a very small amount of radiation, your exposure is much less than if you had a chest X ray or a mammogram or about as much as the amount of "natural" radiation one might receive on an airplane trip across the United States. Experts believe this level to be minimal and safe.

The lumbar spine and the hip are the areas most often targeted in the DXA test. Both areas can be used to represent the rest of the bones in the skeleton and to predict whether you may be at high risk for fractures in other bones. A third area that might be tested is the forearm, just above the wrist. Researchers have shown that this forearm measurement can also be used to help predict a higher risk for fractures in other bones. This test can be done with a machine called peripheral DEXA (pDEXA). It takes only a few minutes and is less expensive to perform than many other measurements.

COMPARATIVE TEST SCORES

After you have been tested, you may want to know how your bone density test score compares to other people of the same age and sex. In the DXA test, your results will include this information, along with the bone density results. The Z-score is data that compares your values with

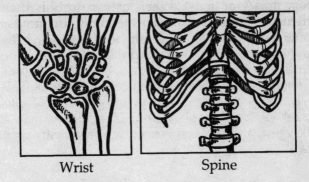

Wrist

Spine

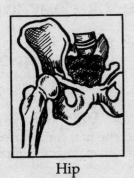

Hip

Figure 3.2—The diagram of the three sites measured in a bone density test.

others your age and sex. But this score is *not* used to make a diagnosis.

QCT (QUANTITATIVE COMPUTED TOMOGRAPHY)

QCT uses a higher amount of radiation to measure the bone density than DXA and takes about ten to twenty-five minutes to complete. It is performed as you lie on a table as you would when an X ray is taken. The test measures the lumbar spine bone density. Recently this test has been adapted by some researchers to measure bone density in the forearm.

There is no pain or discomfort with the QCT. It is accurate and available in most hospitals and larger clinics. The price of QCT is higher than a DXA test, and this test is used less frequently than DXA.

RGA (RADIOGRAPHIC ABSORPTIOMETRY)

RGA takes a standard X ray of the hand and uses computer analysis to estimate bone density. Many areas do not yet have the more sophisticated machinery, such as the DXA, available to measure bone density, and the RGA is a viable way to detect osteoporosis for the masses. Most physicians' offices and clinics have a machine that can be used for this hand X ray, and radiation exposure is minimal and safe.

After the hand X ray is taken, it is sent to a center that calculates the bone density and returns the T-score results to your doctor. The cost of this test ranges from seventy-five to eighty-five dollars. Researchers have shown that this test is accurate and can be used to diagnose osteoporosis.

ULTRASOUND TESTING

The ultrasound test is yet another technique that uses sound waves instead of X rays to estimate bone density. The ultrasound test is frequently performed on your heel bone. It is less expensive than some of the methods described above. While it can be used to predict fracture risk, it is not widely accepted in determining loss of bone in the hip or spine.

More than one type of ultrasound is available for bone density testing. Since the test is simple, relatively low in cost, and does not use radiation, it can be a safe way to complement other types of bone density tests.

URINE TESTS

In those who suffer from osteoporosis, the body is usually very active in breaking down bone. In fact, researchers have discovered that people with this disease are usually working overtime removing bone. A simple urine test (Ostex) is now available that can determine if your body is removing bone rapidly. A positive test result would suggest a higher possibility of osteoporosis.

The test actually measures the amount of bone "breakdown" products removed through the urine. While this urine test may show if your bones have rapid turnover and removal, it does not measure the actual amount of bone that has already been lost or indicate at what stage of osteoporosis the individual may be.

The urine test is also used to tell if the current treatment for osteoporosis is really working. If the test measurement shows that the amount of bone removal drops with medication, then this is a positive sign that the disease is being effectively treated and would suggest a strong likelihood of improvement. These tests may be able to help predict a gain in bone density within a few months of treatment rather than waiting one year for the next bone density test.

NEW TESTS

A recently approved blood test called the Tandem-R Ostase may be used in the future to help doctors find which men and women are at risk for osteoporosis. This test measures a blood marker called *ostase* that monitors the amount of bone turnover in the body. Like the urine test, one benefit of the Tandem-R Ostase is that it can help determine if the correct medication is working within two months of starting treatment.

The traditional bone density tests can only detect changes after bone is built. With the Ostex and Tandem-R Ostase, doctors and patients may know in a shorter period of time whether a given treatment is working. If these tests show no improvement, then another treatment might be considered while there is still time to prevent fractures.

Another test that will be available soon measures the level of zinc in the urine. Studies have shown that elevated levels of zinc in postmenopausal women correlate with decreased bone density (see page 143). These elevated levels of zinc also occur in healthy, younger women in the early stages of menopause and may help doctors estimate who may be at risk for osteoporosis.

REVIEW THE TEST

If you have a bone density test, be sure you review the results with your doctor. He or she can explain what your actual bone strength is and what options you have for prevention or treatment. Use your test results as an early warning sign. It is never too early to take steps for prevention and never too late to treat osteoporosis and prevent fractures.

OTHER CLUES

During recent mass screenings for osteoporosis, researchers found some interesting clues. They realized that women who are *overweight have osteoporosis much less often* than those who are normal or underweight. Researchers also discovered that women who *begin their menstrual periods earlier* in life tend to have a higher bone density than those who happened to begin menstrual periods later. Those women who have an *early menopause* frequently have a lower bone density than those who happen to have a later menopause. We do not know the causes for these findings, but hopefully they will give more clues to solving this mysterious, debilitating disease.

Researchers have found that one measure of the hip on X ray, called *hip axis length*, makes a noticeable difference in a person's risk for fracture. If this length is longer than average, there is often a higher risk, especially in older, white women. It seems that this risk is likely a result of the forces placed on the hip itself because of the shape and length. While we cannot control this risk factor, it may help researchers find better ways to treat and prevent the problem.

Reviewing the following case studies can help give an accurate picture of how specific risk factors, along with increasing age and low bone density scores add up to fractures and disability.

JULIA'S HIP FRACTURE

Seventy-year-old Julia lived alone when she fell and broke her hip. She had been thin most of her adult life, suffered from emphysema and bronchitis, and took prednisone to control her breathing. She had menopause at age forty-four but did not take estrogen therapy and had avoided milk products for most of her life because of resulting diarrhea and stomach cramps. Julia told of her mother being short and stooped over in her later years.

After surgery to repair the broken hip, Julia went to a nearby nursing home for physical therapy. While there, she had a bone density test of her good hip with a resulting T-score of −3.2.

Julia started with calcium and vitamin D supplements, an exercise program, and medications, including Fosamax to try to increase bone strength and lower the chance of future fractures. After one year, Julia's bone density test showed a dramatic increase of 5 percent and her T-score increased to −2.9.

Risk Factors

- Seventy-year-old Caucasian female
- Small stature; underweight

- Chronic obstructive pulmonary disease (COPD)—treated with prednisone for twenty years
- An early menopause at age forty-four with no estrogen treatment
- Lactose intolerance (no dairy products)
- Family history
- Bone density nonfractured hip = 3.2 standard deviations below peak bone mass

CYNTHIA'S ANKLE FRACTURE

Cynthia was fifty-one years old when she tripped over an uneven sidewalk and suffered a painful broken ankle. This slim, Caucasian woman had smoked two packs of cigarettes a day for as long as she could remember, had a hysterectomy at age thirty-three, and did not take estrogen therapy. She also had surgery on her esophagus five years earlier. Cynthia's job as a secretary was sedentary, and she admitted that she had not exercised since her thirties.

After her fracture, a bone density test showed Cynthia's T-score to be −2.9. Her risk of future fractures was abnormally high for a woman in her early fifties.

She immediately began a treatment program for osteoporosis, including calcium, vitamin D, exercise, and stopping cigarettes. She added medication, Miacalcin, which she took daily, and plans to have another bone density scan in about one year.

Risk Factors

- Fifty-one-year-old white female
- Slim build; underweight
- A cigarette smoker (two packs a day)
- An early menopause at thirty-three years old (hysterectomy); no estrogen treatment
- A sedentary job; no exercise program
- Bone density spine = 2.9 standard deviations below peak bone mass

RICHARD'S RIB FRACTURE

Sixty-three-year-old Richard was being treated for emphysema and chronic bronchitis. This two-pack-a-day smoker had taken prednisone for a few weeks at a time over recent years for the bronchitis. Because of his breathing problem, he felt uncomfortable exercising and had a sedentary job as a bank clerk.

During one severe coughing spell, Richard had chest pain and was found to have a fracture of one rib. He had a bone density test, which showed him to be 2.9 standard deviations below normal, a T-score of −2.9.

He began treatment immediately, including removal of risk factors and addition of bone-building medication. After one year, Richard's bone density increased by 4 percent. Today he has a lower risk of fracture than the previous year because of the proactive steps he has taken.

RISK FACTORS

- Sixty-three-year-old Caucasian male
- Normal weight
- A cigarette smoker (two packs a day)
- Chronic obstructive pulmonary disease (COPD); treated with prednisone for twelve years
- A sedentary job; no exercise program
- A history of rib fractures with coughing
- Bone density of hip = 2.9 standard deviations below peak bone mass (T score −2.9)

NIKKI'S ANKLE FRACTURE

At nineteen, Nikki was an energetic and successful competitive gymnast, requiring extensive, constant physical training for more than ten years. She had a very strict diet to prevent weight gain and increase performance, but she had not had a menstrual period in more than one year. While training, Nikki suffered an ankle fracture. Because of her risk factors, she had a bone density test that showed she had actually lost bone strength and was at a higher risk for fractures.

Nikki discussed her situation with her gynecologist, reviewed her diet, added specific hormone replacements, and lightened her training schedule. Since that time, she has had no further fractures.

RISK FACTORS

- Nineteen-year-old Asian female
- Small stature; underweight

- Competitive gymnast for ten years
- Lactose intolerance (no dairy products)
- History of fractures in the ankle
- Loss of menstrual cycle for one year
- Low bone density (low T-score)

DO *NOT* WAIT FOR A FRACTURE

No one has to wait until a fracture occurs. Prevent your first fracture! Using the new methods of testing bone density, along with the breakthrough bone-building medications, every man and woman can enjoy continued mobility and freedom from pain. You can start the easy steps for treatment and prevention of further problems that will allow you to enjoy an active life.

FOUR

Staying Fracture-Free

Staying healthy, active, and fracture-free are optimal goals for everyone, especially as we age. However, to ward off osteoporosis and stay fracture-free, prevention steps are necessary. In millions of people, prevention is possible as groundbreaking reports tell of the importance of calcium, exercise, and estrogen treatment, for post-menopausal women, to keep bones strong.

If you have none or few risk factors and have not been diagnosed with osteoporosis, then the following steps will give a clear understanding of what you can do—starting today—to prevent osteoporosis and stay fracture-free your entire lifetime.

A PREVENTION PROGRAM

1. **Build strong bones with a nutritious diet.**
   Start with calcium. Comprehensive studies show that prevention of osteoporosis should be-

---

Table 4.1
Prevention Steps to Stay Fracture-Free

1. Build strong bones with a nutritious diet—enough calcium.
2. Begin a regular exercise program—weight bearing and back-strengthening.
3. Take estrogen, Fosamax, or other bone-building medication after menopause to prevent bone loss.
4. Stop smoking cigarettes and avoid heavy consumption of alcohol.
5. Educate yourself about medications known to increase risk, especially cortisone products.
6. Be aware of medical problems that increase risk.

---

gin in childhood, while the body is most actively building bone. Adding calcium-rich foods to the diet or supplementing food intake with calcium tablets is a great beginning to build the maximum amount of bone long before age thirty. Some research indicates that our bodies may reach their peak bone mass as young as age sixteen to twenty-five. It makes sense that the stronger our bones are during the teenage and early adult years, the longer they will last when the bone loss begins at midlife.

Childhood. Surprisingly, children need two to four times as much calcium for their body weight as adults. As discussed in Chapter 7, the amount of calcium needed daily for most children to achieve this goal is 500–800 milligrams from diet or calcium supplementation, depending on their age. Use the bone-boosting suggestions in Chapter 7 to guarantee your child's bone health for now and later in life.

Adolescence. Some understanding advice to weight-conscious teenagers is necessary to help ensure they get enough calcium to build strong bones without adding excessive calories to their diets. Giving your family high-calcium but low-fat foods such as skim milk, low-fat milk, low-fat cheeses, nonfat yogurt, and calcium-enriched juices and breads, along with calcium supplements, can make it easy for a weight-conscious teenager to get the necessary 1,500 milligrams of calcium each day.

Young adulthood. Although childhood and adolescent years are crucial for building strong bones, these bone-building measures must continue into adulthood. Young adult women should keep their calcium intake at 1,200 milligrams each day through diet and supplements (see page 127 if you are pregnant), and also remove all possible risk factors that are within your control. Remember that the gradual process of bone removal can begin as early as age thirty, even though your bones are still strong and you show no signs of disease.

Menopause. It is not too late to keep bones strong in later adult years, though many women begin to experience fractures shortly after menopause due to the drastic decline of estrogen and the injurious result on bone mass. After this life change, women should increase their calcium intake to 1,500 milligrams each day through diet and supplements. An average calcium diet after menopause only contains about 800 milligrams of calcium. In fact, studies have shown that 80 percent of all postmenopausal women do not get adequate calcium to stop bone loss.

In women and men over age sixty-five, one recent study found fewer fractures and better bone density in those who took calcium and vitamin D supplements.

Along with adding more calcium to the diet, it is vital to keep the other controllable risk factors in check. If you have more than two or three of the risk factors discussed in Chapter 2, talk with your doctor about having a bone density test to see if other treatment is needed.

Add vitamin D. Vitamin D is also necessary to prevent osteoporosis. It helps the intestine absorb calcium and phosphorus into the bones and teeth, making them stronger and helping to guard against fractures. Most children get enough vitamin D in their fortified milk, which contains 100 IU (international units) of vitamin D per eight-ounce glass. Still, 100 IU is only one fourth of the 400 IU daily requirement needed to build strong bones.

While it is estimated that about fifteen minutes of sun exposure may allow the body to produce vitamin D, the newer sunscreens can block the rays that the body needs to make vitamin D. Especially in adults, working indoors, weather conditions, and other factors can make it impossible to get vitamin D from sun exposure.

Older adults, especially those in nursing homes, do not get enough sun exposure for adequate vitamin D production, and they only have half the ability to convert sunlight into vitamin D that a twenty-year-old does. Use the specific suggestions in Chapter 8 to make sure you are receiving enough vitamin D to protect your bones.

2. **Begin a regular exercise program.**

Calcium, by itself, is limited in building bone unless it is combined with a consistent exercise program. Such a program must include weight-bearing exercises, plus exercises that strengthen the muscles of the back and legs. While calcium helps to build bone, weight-bearing exercises such as walking, biking, low-impact aerobics, tennis, stair-climbing, and rowing all stimulate bone-building cells to do their work. Remember, researchers have found that stronger back muscles can mean stronger bones, too.

Patients who for medical reasons are unable to walk, and even healthy, young astronauts who are weightless in space, have all been shown to lose bone. Exercise and movement are the keys to building stronger bones while staying fracture-free. Follow the instructions in Chapter 6 as you begin a regular exercise program to ward off fractures.

3. **Take estrogen, Fosamax, or other bone-building medication after menopause to prevent bone loss.**

For women, the single most effective prevention for osteoporosis is to take estrogen replacement therapy (ERT) after menopause. When menopause occurs earlier than the usual age of forty-five to fifty-five, the risk of fractures increases. Also, if both ovaries are removed by surgery before the time of menopause, then the risk is higher.

At the time of menopause, every woman should decide with her doctor whether she will add estrogen. If taken within the first few years after menopause, this can prevent or at least greatly delay osteoporosis. Many experts advise taking estrogen to prevent osteoporosis, unless a specific reason such as a family history of breast cancer might make it dangerous. But since experts don't always agree, talk with your doctor to decide what is best for your own situation.

The most common estrogen used for prevention and treatment is *conjugated estrogen*, which is only available by prescription. (See page 80 for some of most commonly used estrogens.) The dose of estrogen needed to prevent and treat osteoporosis is the equivalent of 0.625 milligrams conjugated estrogen daily. This amount is given for twenty-one to twenty-five days each month beginning the first day of the month.

Progestin, another hormone, is added around days sixteen to twenty-one each month. This hormone reduces the constant stimulation of the lining of the uterus by estrogen that can cause irregular bleeding and increase the risk of developing endometrial cancer. There are also combination treatments available that use estrogen and progestin combined in one tablet given daily throughout the month.

If your menopause was natural, without surgery, then estrogen treatment can lead to bleeding from the vagina, since it replaces the estrogen that helped cause menstrual periods earlier in life. This bleeding may be regular or there may be spotting. The good news is that some studies show about *80 percent* of women who receive estrogen replacement therapy (ERT) or the combination of estrogen and progestin do *not* have bleeding after one year.

The risk of cancer of the uterus is slightly increased during estrogen treatment. This is easily managed if you will see your doctor on a regular basis to be sure no other problems develop. A simple test called an *endometrial biopsy* can be done in your doctor's office to check the lining of the uterus and be sure there are no abnormal causes of bleeding. Of course, if you have had a hysterectomy, you will not have to worry about vaginal bleeding from estrogen, and the dose of estrogen is the same.

RISKS INVOLVED

With ERT there is a small increase in risk of gallstones, fluid retention, and headache. Check with your doctor if you notice any new problems. Some researchers have also found a slight increased risk of breast cancer with estrogen treatment. Some women may already be at higher than normal risk, such as those who have a family member with breast cancer. If you've had breast cancer, most experts would advise against ERT. Weigh the benefits and also the risks of ERT, then decide with your doctor whether estrogen is a safe course of treatment. Of course, regular self-examination, mammogram, and follow-up with your doctor should be continued for all women.

An added benefit is that estrogen treatment can also lower the risk of heart attack and other cardiovascular disease by 40 percent. Newer studies suggest that estrogen may even help stave off Alzheimer's disease.

There are usually more bonuses than problems with estrogen replacement after menopause unless you have specific reasons, such as a personal or family history of breast cancer. The argument in favor of estrogen is strong when it can lower the risk of osteoporosis, along with greatly lowering the risk of heart disease.

After menopause, estrogen can be taken indefinitely, but it appears that when estrogen is stopped, bone density may diminish and protection against fractures drops.

When estrogen treatment is taken to prevent or treat osteoporosis, it cannot be stopped without losing protection against fractures. Research has shown that of estrogen prescriptions given, 20 to 30 percent may not be refilled, 35 to 40 percent of persons do not return for refills, and after three years, 75 to 80 percent of patients no longer are taking the medication.

The reason for stopping estrogen may include worries about side effects, concern about bleeding brought on by the treatment, or lack of knowledge of the possible benefits. Improved education about the benefits and risks may help, but some women and physicians may still have concerns about long-term estrogen treatment.

The evidence is that estrogen treatment to prevent fractures of the hips and other bones after menopause and to lower the risk of heart attack may outweigh the risks in many but not all women. We've already discussed the perilous risk of a broken hip, which can lead to an early death.

As with all medications you must compare the benefits and risks of taking estrogen after menopause in your own situation. If you decide ERT is too risky, consider alternative medications such as Fosamax, Evista, Didronel, or Miacalcin.

For example, for women who are not able to take estrogen because of previous breast cancer, Fosamax is effective in preventing bone loss after menopause in 86 percent of cases. This means that 86 percent of women who take Fosamax for prevention of bone loss in menopause will maintain their bone strength, about the same as with estrogen treatment. With Fosamax there will be no cardiovascular risk reduction and no effects of estrogen.

Your physician can help you decide if Fosamax, Evista, or other breakthrough medications should be considered when estrogen treatment is not chosen.

4. **Stop smoking cigarettes and avoid heavy consumption of alcohol.**

   Stopping cigarettes and cutting back on alcohol are prevention measures you hold in your own hands—literally! In fact, the risk of osteoporosis drops in half when you stop smoking. The chances of having heart disease, cancer, stroke, and emphysema also decrease upon quitting.

   Stopping smoking is not easy. Yet if you are concerned about your bone health, as well as your overall health, call your local American Lung Association about programs to help you quit. Likewise, cutting back on alcohol, if you are a heavy drinker, will not be an easy task. Talk with your doctor about both of these "bone-robbing" habits and ask for a referral to organizations that can offer support. Chapter 9 has more information on smoking and heavy alcohol consumption and the connection with bone loss.

5. **Educate yourself about medications known to increase risk.**

Some medications can greatly increase the risk of osteoporosis. Probably the most common are the *cortisone-type* drugs. Not only are these drugs necessary and lifesaving, but they are used to manage very serious illnesses. For example, cortisone-type drugs can make breathing easier for a person with asthma, chronic bronchitis, emphysema, and other respiratory problems. While each person is different, the unwanted side effect of osteoporosis is usually dependent on how much cortisone is taken and the length of treatment. The longer it is given and the higher the dose, the more severe the osteoporosis is likely to be.

Prednisone is the most commonly used cortisone-type drug. While most doctors try to use the lowest possible dose for the shortest length of time to keep the side effects to a minimum, this is not always possible, depending on the seriousness of the disease being treated. If you must take prednisone, be sure you remove all other risk factors for osteoporosis (take calcium supplements, exercise, and stop smoking cigarettes). Medications including estrogen and Fosamax can be added to prevent loss. If you need to be on prednisone for a length of time, it may be a good idea to have a bone density test to be sure osteoporosis is not present before you start taking prednisone.

There are some ways to make prednisone as

safe as possible if you must take this medication. The American College of Rheumatology guidelines suggest a bone density test at the start of prednisone treatment. This can help determine whether you are already in some danger of low bone density.

The guidelines also suggest that those who must take prenisone over a long period of time be sure to take 1,500 milligrams of calcium through diet and supplements each day. You should also take 800 units of vitamin D.

The guidelines further stress removing all possible risk factors to minimize the chance of osteoporosis while on this treatment. This would include a regular exercise program, avoiding cigarettes, and avoiding excess alcohol, as discussed in Chapter 2. Estrogen treatment for women past menopause and even oral contraceptives can be considered for younger women who must take prednisone. Fosamax and Evista are now available for those women who do not take estrogen. Men should be tested to make certain their testosterone levels are normal.

After six to twelve months, it may be a good idea to have another bone density test to make sure the prednisone or other cortisone product has not caused bone loss. Keeping a regular check on bone density during your cortisone treatment will enable you to stop bone loss when you get the first signs.

Short courses of treatment with cortisone drugs, especially at low doses, are not very dangerous. These doses are used in short bursts in cases of mild or acute asthma, bursitis, skin rashes, and other problems. Also, cortisone drugs can be given by injection into a joint in arthritis, or for problems such as tendinitis. These injections offer quick and effective relief and do not raise the risk of osteoporosis.

Antacids are another type of medication that can increase your risk of osteoporosis. While we all take these at some time for quick relief for an acid stomach, if taken in high doses, some antacids can cause a loss of bone. The specific bone-robbing antacids contain aluminum and cause an excessive loss of calcium from the body. Our bodies then begin to remove calcium in bones to replace the loss. A higher supplement of calcium may offset the extra calcium loss if you must take these antacids.

While *thyroid medication* is essential for those who have an underactive thyroid, if too much thyroid medication is taken, or if the thyroid itself is overactive, osteoporosis and fractures will result. At times, even what would be considered correct amounts of thyroid treatment can result in osteoporosis. Your doctor can monitor this periodically with a simple blood test and give you advice on various thyroid medication doses.

Some of the medications used for *seizures* such as Dilantin (phenytoin) can also increase the chance of osteoporosis. The risks can be reduced and the medication can be continued if a few preventive steps are taken. It is a good idea to review your medication history with your doctor and see if this might increase the chance of osteoporosis. If it does, start prevention measures to ward off fractures.

6. **Be aware of medical problems that can increase risk.**

Some medical problems increase the chance of osteoporosis. For example, *rheumatoid arthritis*, which affects 1 to 2 percent of the population with painful joint swelling, definitely increases the chance of osteoporosis. These patients also often take prednisone, are less active, and are often underweight, adding even more serious risk factors for fractures.

The added risk of rheumatoid arthritis is strong enough that it is included in the score self-test for osteoporosis on page 27. The higher risk can be managed by removing any other risk factors, when possible, and by getting your bone density test. If your bone density is lower than normal, be careful to take steps to preserve or even increase your bone strength.

Chronic lung disease, mainly *chronic bronchitis* and *emphysema* from smoking cigarettes, also raises the chance of osteoporosis to higher levels. Some of the medications used to treat these diseases also increase the risk. Removing controllable risk factors is vital, including stopping cigarettes, which is important for your overall health. Be sure to have your bone density measured so you can take proper steps when needed to prevent or treat osteoporosis.

Diabetes mellitus and some *intestinal problems*, including those that require surgery for removal of part of the stomach, may increase the chance of osteoporosis. If any of these problems affect you, try to remove other risk factors to prevent osteoporosis. Again, stay on top of your bone density measurement for an accurate analysis. This will allow you to start treatment before a fracture happens.

FIVE

New Bone-Building Treatments and Other Ways to Prevent Fractures

Treatment for osteoporosis is easy and effective once you know that a problem exists. For example, I recently saw Sandra, an executive with a large insurance company. Her mother had fallen, breaking her hip, and was now in a long-term care facility for recovery. Seeing how helpless her mother had become from this break, Sandra wanted to know if she was also at risk for osteoporosis and the subsequent fractures.

Although she had begun menopause at age fifty, she chose not to take estrogen replacement therapy (ERT). After a bone density test, Sandra discovered that she was in Stage 2 and was likely to increase her risk of fractures over the next few years unless something was done immediately. This lifesaving information allowed her to begin a treatment program years earlier than if she had waited for the first fracture. And she may prevent having a fracture altogether because of the early treatment and intervention.

Of course, prevention is the best way to avoid fractures. However, for the more than thirty million people in the United States who have osteoporosis, treatment is still effective in staying fracture-free and must be started immediately.

If you have osteoporosis, you may wonder if this treatment, including new medications that actually build bone, really works. The answer is a resounding yes! If you have a fracture from osteoporosis or if you have been diagnosed with osteoporosis before having a fracture, treatment entails the following steps.

Table 5.1
Treatment Steps to Halt Osteoporosis and Fractures

1. **Start the prevention steps listed in Chapter 4, including:**

   - Build strong bones with a nutritious diet, especially added calcium and vitamin D.
   - Begin a regular exercise program.
   - Take estrogen after menopause to prevent bone loss.
   - Stop smoking cigarettes and avoid heavy consumption of alcohol.
   - Educate yourself about medications known to increase risk (i.e., corticosteroids and antacids containing aluminum, among many.)
   - Be aware of medical problems that can increase risk.

2. **Start on breakthrough medications to increase bone density.**
3. **Prevent falls.**
4. **Try safe, alternative treatment.**

A TREATMENT PROGRAM

1. **Start the prevention steps listed in Chapter 4.**

   Reread Chapter 4, if needed, to fully comprehend the important measures you must take to keep your bones strong. A diet with enough calcium and vitamin D, regular weight-bearing and strengthening exercises, and estrogen replacement therapy if you are a postmenopausal woman, are all key factors in building strong bones and preventing further bone loss and fractures. Along with these preventive measures, remove all risk factors over which you have control. We thoroughly discuss risk factors in Chapter 2, and you should be able to indentify those which pertain to you.

   Now let's move to the next treatment steps, which are vital to preventing further bone loss and future fractures; some can actually make your bones stronger.

2. **Start on the breakthrough medications to build bone density.**

   Medications are crucial for improving bone density after osteoporosis has been diagnosed. Today there are four basic groups of medications to consider if you have bone loss, including estrogen, bisphosphonates, calcitonin, and fluoride.

ESTROGEN

As explained in Chapter 4, estrogen is still the most effective prevention for osteoporosis after menopause, as it efficiently replaces the hormone made by the ovaries before menopause. It is well known that estrogen treatment within the first few years of menopause can delay or even prevent the progress of osteoporosis. There is about an 85 percent chance that with estrogen you will prevent bone loss in menopause.

Besides excellent prevention, estrogen is now widely used to treat osteoporosis. In fact, estrogen treatment has been proven to increase bone density. Some researchers have found as much as a *5 percent* increase in bone density in patients who took estrogen. This increase can prevent further fractures. Without treatment, it is very common for women to lose *1 to 3 percent* bone density each year after menopause. But remember that for fracture protection you must continue taking estrogen.

Don't forget that the *low bone density/fracture connection* is strong—even stronger than the *high blood cholesterol/heart attack connection*. If low bone density improves, the risk of fracture is reduced. Estrogen is one medication that can improve bone density and lower fracture risk even if osteoporosis is already present.

Since every person is different, consider talking to your doctor to see if you should add estrogen treatment. If you have had breast cancer, have a family member who has had breast cancer, or if you have had blood clots (thrombophlebitis), blood clot in the lung (pulmonary embolus), heart attack, or severe headaches, then let your doctor advise you for your own situation. Every woman on estrogen should have regular checkups to control the slightly higher risk of uterine cancer associated with this treatment.

Another benefit in estrogen treatment is its excellent effect on cardiovascular disease. For example, estrogen treatment usually lowers the risk of heart attack by *40 percent*. In fact, research has not reported a higher risk of death overall in women who take estrogens after menopause.

BONE-BUILDING BISPHOSPHONATES

The bisphosphonates are the newest group of medications that improve bone density. Unlike estrogen, these medications are not hormones. Instead, bisphosphonates work to build bone by slowing the removal of bone while allowing more bone to be formed. Thus the total amount of bone is increased. These breakthrough medications can be used to prevent osteoporosis and for treatment to prevent fractures after the diagnosis of osteoporosis has been made.

Fosamax for Treatment

Fosamax (alendronate) and Didronel (etidronate) are two of the biphosphonates available at this time. Fosamax has been approved by the United

Table 5.2
Medications Used to Stop Bone Loss

BRAND NAMES	GENERIC NAMES
Fosamax	Alendronate
Premarin, Estrace, Estratab, Estraderm	Estrogen
Didronel	Etidronate
Evista	Raloxifene
Miacalcin	Calcitonin

States Food and Drug Administration (FDA) for use in the prevention and treatment of osteoporosis. Through test after test, this breakthrough medication has been shown to significantly increase bone density. Studies with Fosamax show *more than 90 percent* of patients respond to treatment with this medication. Over a one- to three-year period, people on this medication have had increases in bone density of *6 percent* or more. Studies also show Fosamax increases bone density over *9 percent* after 5 years.

Because low bone density is strongly connected to increased risk for fractures, scientists have realized that as bone density improves, the risk of fractures drops. In fact, studies in postmenopausal women showed a drop in the rate of hip fractures by *50 percent* in women who took Fosamax. This improved rate of hip fracture is important in older persons with osteoporosis because of the increased risk of death and loss of independence after this particular injury.

More revealing studies have found a drop in the rate of fractures in the spine by about *50 percent* and about *30 percent* fewer fractures in the wrist and shoulder. This reduction in fractures is crucial as these small cracks in the vertebrae cause loss of height and create the stooped upper back known as dowager's hump. Studies with Fosamax have shown that it reduces the likelihood of loss of height and stooped-over posture in women with osteoporosis after menopause. This major benefit offers new hope to millions as it might help to prevent outward signs of the disease. Recent studies show that Fosamax reduces fractures by almost half in the first year after it is begun.

The beneficial effect of bone-building using Fosamax appears to continue over at least five years. The drug is still so new that doctors have not yet determined how long the medication should be continued. Some researchers feel that if the bone density improves enough to return to a low risk for fracture, then stopping the medication temporarily may be acceptable. Then bone density should be checked periodically to make sure the measurement does not drop. Your doctor can guide you.

Can estrogen be combined with Fosamax for treatment of osteoporosis? Studies are being completed which show the effect of combined treatment in treating osteoporosis. Discuss your situation with your doctor.

A newer use for Fosamax includes a lower dose at five milligrams daily for *prevention of osteoporosis* in those women who are at higher risk after menopause but are not able to take estrogen. It is used along with other prevention measures and given around 85 percent chance of preventing bone loss.

Precautions

Most persons who take Fosamax have no side effects. Because it is not easily absorbed, it should be taken on an empty stomach with an eight-ounce glass of water. After you take the 5- or 10-milligram tablet, do not eat any food or drink any beverage for thirty to sixty minutes to enhance absorption. Coffee or orange juice can lower the absorption of Fosamax by *40 percent*.

It is also important not to lie down for thirty to sixty minutes after you take Fosamax. This usually prevents symptoms of esophageal irritation: indigestion, heartburn, or abdominal discomfort. If you have had esophageal problems or difficulty swallowing, it is wise to first check with your doctor to be sure Fosamax can be tolerated. If you notice heartburn, indigestion, or other digestive problems when taking the medication, let your doctor know.

Didronel

Didronel (etidronate) is available for treatment of osteoporosis, yet it is not formally approved by the U.S. Food and Drug Administration. Some studies have shown an increase in bone density with Didronel in women with osteoporosis after menopause, increasing from *1 to 6 percent* over three years in some patients. Like Fosamax, Didronel works to increase bone density by slowing the bone-removal process. Some researchers have found that with this medication the bone building slows down or levels out after two to three years.

Didronel is given for two weeks at a time, then stopped. It is repeated in about thirteen weeks. Didronel is taken in this way because taking it daily can limit bone building, as well as bone removal. You may think that this is an unusual way to take any medication; however, most patients fit it into their schedule by marking their calendars.

Precautions

Like Fosamax, Didronel is not absorbed easily in the stomach, so you should take it with a full glass of water and not eat or drink for two hours after taking this medication. Most patients do not have side effects from Didronel, but the most frequent include nausea and diarrhea.

CALCITONIN

Calcitonin is another medication available to treat osteoporosis. One of its actions is to help slow bone removal, which should make the bone density improve. It has also been used immediately after spinal fractures because patients find it gives some pain relief.

Calcitonin is a hormone (but not estrogen) and is available as an injection (Calcimar) and as a nasal spray (Miacalcin). The injection is an older form of the medicine and is taken two to three times a week. The nasal spray has been more popular with patients than the injection and is taken daily, alternating right and left nostrils each day.

Calcitonin is indicated for osteoporosis in women more than five years after menopause. Most clinicians feel it is especially useful in those who cannot or choose not to take estrogen or Fosamax.

Researchers have found that in postmenopausal women with osteoporosis, calcitonin increases bone density, especially in the spine. Some have found that Miacalcin (the nasal spray) increased bone density, especially the first year, but had less effect the second year of treatment. It is possible that future studies will show that with continued Miacalcin treatment, the chance of fracture from osteoporosis will be lower.

PRECAUTIONS

Most patients do not have side effects from the injection or nasal spray form of calcitonin, although the injection may cause nausea, feelings of flushing, tingling, or other problems. These feelings are not usually a problem with Miacalcin, yet some patients report feeling irritation of the nasal lining (rhinitis).

FLUORIDE

Fluoride has been used for years in osteoporosis but is not yet approved for treatment by the U.S. FDA. Years ago, scientists noted that women who lived in areas with higher fluoride content in drinking water had fewer fractures. When fluoride was first tried as a treatment, higher doses were found to cause many side effects. Lately, lower doses have been used that reduce the side effects, while also improving bone density. These forms of fluoride are more well tolerated and may be used in the future, especially as a supplement to one of the other newer medications.

Table 5.3
Bone-Building Medications—Brand Names

ESTROGENS
Estraderm
Estrace
Estratab
Premarin

BISPHOSPHONATES
Fosamax
*Didronel**

SELECTIVE ESTROGEN
Evista

CALCITONINS
Miacalcin
Calcimar

FLUORIDE*

Not yet approved by the U.S. FDA for use in osteoporosis.

Both increased bone formation and greater bone density result from fluoride treatment. However, it has not been shown to convincingly lower the chance of fractures. Interestingly, some researchers have found more fractures in certain cases with fluoride.

Nevertheless, there are new types of fluoride treatments awaiting approval by the Food and Drug Administration at this time. For example, a slow-release fluoride in combination with calcium has been found to strengthen bones and prevent spinal fractures in women with osteoporosis. Slow-release fluoride avoids the toxic effects of higher fluoride doses and has been effective in women with mild to moderate bone loss.

Evista (raloxifene) is one of a new group of medications used to build bone in osteoporosis. This group of medicines was actually developed to block the effect of estrogens in breast cancer and is called "anti-estrogen." Raloxifene does not increase the risk of breast cancer, which is one of the reasons many women don't take estrogen after menopause. It also does not cause uterine bleeding and irregular menstrual periods, which can happen with estrogen treatment. The irregular menstrual bleeding is another major reason that many women don't keep up their estrogen treatment. If estrogen is stopped, the benefits of osteoporosis protection stop as well.

Evista can provide the benefits of estrogen replacement treatment for the bones in prevention and treatment of osteoporosis and does not cause breast tenderness. It may also lower blood cholesterol as a beneficial side effect. Evista does not help reduce hot flashes.

Several medications in this group are being developed and may be available over the next few years as research continues.

3. Prevent falls.

Preventing falls is a crucial step in treating osteoporosis. Whether from a weakness in the legs, knees, or hips, the chance of falling greatly increases with advancing age. For those in Stage 3 or 4, one fall can result in a hip fracture, hospitalization, surgery, and even death. Other physical problems can complicate these falls. These problems range from unsteadiness, thinning bones, or weakness in muscles to dizziness, heart problems, and medications that cause disorientation.

Studies show that each year *more than one third of all people over age sixty-five fall at least once*. Falling can push an elderly person with osteoporosis into self-imposed immobility, dependence, and even depression.

It makes sense that if bones are thin from osteoporosis, then less severe stress is needed to cause a fracture. Sometimes problems that cause falls and injuries are difficult to identify; sometimes a fall is simply bad luck. However, tripping over furniture, telephone cords, rugs, and outdoor hoses at home can be avoided. Good lighting, especially for nighttime, may result in fewer falls and limit this risk factor.

Some problems are easier to control, such as a thorough understanding of the possible side effects of medications. For example, some medications for hypertension can cause dizziness. Tranquilizers and sleeping pills can cause unsteadiness. Alcohol can make you unsteady and careless.

Simple preventive measures make avoiding falls almost effortless. For example, you can avoid slipping on smooth floors if proper shoes are worn. Shoes should be well fitted with rubber or gripper soles, and smooth floors should not be waxed.

Installing new and brighter lighting in your home, especially in doorways, hallways, and stairways, can help you avoid falling. And if necessary, purchasing assistive devices, such as a cart to move larger items around the house, grab bars by your bathtub and toilet, and safety strips to anchor rugs or carpeting, can make the living environment safer for those who are fearful of falling. Look at the following tips to prevent falls:

- **Tip #1: Check your vision.** Impaired vision increases the risk of falls and fractures. Be sure to get regular eye examinations, and wear corrective lenses, if needed.
- **Tip #2: Use a cane or walker for steadiness.** If you are unsteady walking, a cane or walker can be a lifesaver. Canes or walkers can be very useful in helping to steady your balance, especially in bad weather or with slick floors. Be sure to use the cane in the hand opposite the painful hip or knee and keep it by the bedside for when you need to get up at night.
- **Tip #3: Improve safety measures in your home.** It is important to thoroughly check the home for any obstacles that may hinder walking or cause someone to trip and fall. This would include tattered or frayed rugs, telephone or electrical cords, furniture in commonly used pathways, or uneven tiles or wood flooring. An easy way to fall-proof a home is to have a relative or friend walk through the home to check for hazards. You would be surprised at the number of fall-related injuries we treat in our clinic that are the result of patients tripping on electrical cords. Take precautionary measures: Make sure floors are not overly waxed or slippery. Use double-sided tape or safety strips to secure the edges of area rugs. Make sure electrical and phone cords are tucked behind furniture or out of the main walkway. A portable phone avoids long cords.

Remove any clutter, debris, or throw rugs that could cause a fall. Check to make sure your flooring is even throughout the house, and make repairs to the uneven places that could cause a potential hazard. Personal alarm buttons worn around the neck can bring quick assistance when needed.

- **Tip #4: Make sure lighting is adequate.** Lighting is another fall factor over which you have control. Many people have not taken a critical look at the lighting in their home for years. Especially as we age, we need two to three times as much illumination as a younger person. Check the lightbulbs and replace low-wattage bulbs, if necessary. Proper lighting at night is especially important. Since many people get up at night due to sleep problems, get a night-light, or several. You should definitely have one in the bathroom. A flashlight beside the bed can also be helpful.

- **Tip #5: Install safety bars in the bathroom.** The bathroom is a common place for a fall, and is especially dangerous because of the hard tile surfaces. Many older adults feel dizzy or lightheaded when they stand up quickly. Some stand up from the toilet seat and are overcome by dizziness, resulting in a fall and subsequent injuries. If there are safety "grab bars" around the toilet, tub, and shower, or on a wall nearby, the chance of falling greatly diminishes. These bars are simple to install and are available in most home supply stores. A rubber mat for the tub or shower also increases safety.

- **Tip #6: Use a wheelchair if unsteady when walking.** If you are limited by hip or knee pain from a previous fracture, you may need a wheel-chair. It may not be necessary for daily use at home or even short shopping trips, but do not hesitate to borrow or rent a wheelchair or power scooter when a longer trip or sight-seeing is planned. It is something to consider seriously when the alternative is missing out on the trip or event.

4. Try safe, alternative treatment.

While traditional medical treatments afford many lifesaving and life-extending therapies, millions of people have found additional im-provement with alternative or complementary treatments. This multifaceted approach includes using measures such as exercise, diet, relaxa-tion, herbal therapy, and biofeedback, among others. For example, Chinese tai chi has been found to reduce the risk of fracture in older adults as it helps develop flexibility and bal-ance. A diet high in calcium, vitamins, minerals, and soy foods is crucial prevention and treat-ment of osteoporosis for all ages. Therapeutic massage can help to loosen stiff muscles, and exercise is an important factor in building stronger bone.

The following complementary measures are just a few types of treatments you may consider in a comprehensive program to beat osteopo-rosis.

CHIROPRACTIC

While some consider chiropractic treatment to be alternative, this drug-free approach to healing is well established. Chiropractic relies on manipulation of the spine and muscles, in conjunction with nutrition and exercise. Doctors of chiropractic are unique in that instead of treating specific symptoms, they are primarily interested in realigning the spinal bones, which chiropractors believe are dislodged from their normal healthy alignment due to stress, trauma, or other causes.

Spinal manipulation or adjustment attempts to relieve pain by increasing the mobility between spinal vertebrae that have become restricted or locked or out of position. The manipulations can be gentle stretching or pressure, repeated minor motions, or a few high-velocity thrusts.

Doctors of chiropractic (DC) are licensed by each state and must complete two years of undergraduate study, along with a four-year course at a chiropractic college.

MASSAGE AND THERAPEUTIC TOUCH

Therapeutic touch affects the body as a whole. This form of drug-free therapy has been shown to increase circulation, give relief from musculoskeletal pain and tension, act as a mind/body form of stress release, increase flexibility, and increase mobility.

Massage of the muscles of the back give relief to sore muscles and help exercises. Find a licensed massage therapist—health spas, gyms, and physicians' and chiropractic offices often have massage therapists available.

The American Massage Therapy Association provides a national referral service for qualified, professional massage therapists. Some licensed physical therapists and registered nurses now practice massage therapy, as well.

ACUPUNCTURE

Acupuncture is a form of hyperstimulation for pain or symptom relief that has been approved by the Food and Drug Administration as a medical device. Researchers cannot explain how or why it works but have increasing evidence that there may be a physiological explanation for the therapy.

Relief from acupuncture is experienced through certain reflexes in the body that occur by way of the nervous system. By stimulating one part of the body and using pathways of the nervous system, an effect is obtained in the same or other portion of the body. Additionally, it is believed that acupuncture causes the body to release endorphins—the body's own pain-relieving chemicals—which may add to the feeling of relaxation. Some studies even suggest that acupuncture may trigger the release of certain neural hormones including serotonin, which adds to the feeling of calmness.

If you try acupuncture, do so with your doctor's approval, and ask for a referral to a *licensed* practitioner who uses only disposable needles. Generally you will go through a series of at least eight to ten treatments before making a decision about the treatment's efficacy. You may not feel any relief or it may give extremely long-lasting relief.

Acupuncture has very few contraindications, and the side effects are minimal; however, certain disorders, such as easy bleeding and local infection, may preclude you from receiving this treatment.

BIOFEEDBACK

Biofeedback is a relaxation technique that uses electrical devices to measure such body responses as heart rate and muscle contractions. This type of therapy is based on the idea that when people are given information about their body's internal processes, they can use this information to learn to control those processes. It requires you to be connected to a machine that informs you and your therapist when you are physically relaxing your body. With sensors placed over specific muscle sites, the therapist will read the tension in your muscles, heart rate, breathing pattern, sweat produced, or body temperature. Any one or all of these readings can let the trained biofeedback therapist know if you are learning to relax.

The ultimate goal of biofeedback is to use this skill outside the therapist's office when you are facing real stressors. When successful, electronic biofeedback can help you control your heart rate, blood pressure, breathing patterns, and muscle tension when you are *not* hooked up to the machine. Some therapists recommend relaxation tapes for patients to have relaxation techniques at home.

HOMEOPATHIC MEDICINE

Homeopathy is a therapeutic system of medicine developed in the late eighteenth century. It is based on the principle of "like cures like symptom." In other words, remedies that would cause a potential problem in large doses will actually encourage the body to heal more rapidly if given in small doses.

Homeopathic remedies are highly diluted formulas of plant, mineral, and animal substances that can produce symptoms of a particular ailment in healthy people but alleviate similar symptoms in a sick person. The idea is to stimulate the body's immune reaction to throw off the offender.

Though homeopathic remedy sales are rapidly growing (25 percent increase in 1995 and 1996, according to the National Center for Homeopathy), this type of alternative medical treatment has always been scrutinized by the Western medical community. If you seek advice from a homeopathic practitioner, be sure to ask for credentials. Where did he or she study homeopathy? Did she pass a certification exam?

HEALING FOODS AND HERBS

According to the World Health Organization, 80 percent of the earth's population uses plant remedies. For example, the herbs horsetail and suma are recommended by some to help in osteoporosis. While suma appears to affect the sexual function of men and women, horsetail is said to facilitate the use of calcium in the body, aiding the development of strong bones and nails.

Because many herbal preparations are not regulated by the Food and Drug Administration (FDA), you cannot be sure that you are getting a pure form. Often herbs can affect your response to prescribed medication or may even be toxic. Therefore, it is imperative to speak with your doctor or nutritionist before taking herbs to make sure that the product will not cause you any harm.

Perhaps the most important element gaining success with mind/body interplay is the placebo effect or a belief that treatment will work. This approach to wellness demands your personal involvement and commitment to improved health as you learn and perform the various modes of therapy along with continuing prescribed medications. Most important, using the mind/body modes of treatment forces you to be in touch with your body and your emotions and to listen to them. In many cases, simply understanding your body, your illness, and the accompanying symptoms will help you ward off a serious problem as you take action *before* a crisis occurs.

SIX

Use 'Em or Lose 'Em!

You would never miss a workout again if you took to heart the wealth of scientific evidence that points to exercise as a *key player* in staving off osteoporosis. As discussed in Chapter 2, starting a regular exercise program is one important risk factor for the disease that you can control. While you cannot change your sex, age, or family history, you can change your exercise habits. Not only does exercise help to keep bones strong, it strengthens the muscles, gives the joints more support, and keeps you limber, which can help in preventing falls. For those who exercise regularly, it may shorten the time of recovery and decrease pain, if they do experience a fracture.

Some revealing studies have shown that a marked decrease in physical activity, such as being confined to bed rest, results in profound decline in bone mass. A prime example of this is seen in the bone disorders of astronauts. Tests on those who experience weightlessness show the necessity of physical activity in keeping bones strong.

Interestingly, too much physical activity can also result in bone disorders. The hormonal imbalances from intense exercise and diet control can lead to decreased bone mass, osteoporosis, and fractures. This is commonly experienced among competitive female athletes. Balancing exercise and postinjury recovery time is crucial to stopping osteoporosis.

After age forty, many of us become less active due to more sedentary work. This type of lifestyle is even more common in those over age fifty, and worse yet, other risk factors, such as osteoarthritis or heart disease, may further limit physical activity. Planning periods of physical activity throughout the day may be necessary during midlife and later to maintain bone strength and flexibility.

While many of my patients opt to join the group of weekend warriors who work sedentary jobs for five days, then use Saturday or Sunday to catch up on their exercise, it appears that regular, daily activity is much more beneficial for bone health. Studies from the State University of New York show that postmenopausal women who walk one hour longer *per day* than other women have stronger, thicker bones in their hips—bone mass comparable to women four years younger.

Exercise does not have to be excessive or strenuous to stop or reverse bone loss. Two studies involving more than eight hundred older adults found that those who walked the equivalent of at least twenty to thirty minutes per day had much denser bones than inactive adults. Numerous studies have made similar conclusions—weight-bearing exercise, such as walking, can stimulate bone mass to stay strong in premenopausal, postmenopausal, and elderly women. If you happen to be a man, do not think that this lets you off the hook. It is certain to do the same for men of all ages!

For some of us, regular exercise is already an important part of our busy, health-conscious lifestyle. However, the reality is that many of us have ignored recommendations from health professionals to stay active and will be faced with the painful, debilitating results in the future—fractures and immobility from osteoporosis.

AGING WELL

The Centers for Disease Control reports that nearly four out of five adults in America get almost no exercise at all. Possibly as a consequence of that, *40 percent* of all Americans older than seventy-five are unable to walk even two blocks, according to the National Institute on Aging. Nearly *32 percent* are unable to climb stairs, and 22 *percent* cannot lift ten pounds. Obviously, aging well and staying fracture-free depend on regular exercise and activity.

Weight-bearing exercises, specifically walking, aerobics, racket sports, and strenuous strength training, are crucial to increasing bone mass. This type of activity puts vertical force on the bones. This force creates mini electrical currents that help to strengthen the bone being stressed.

Based on the most recent findings to date, strength training is also an important aid in the prevention and reversal of osteoporosis. Women, especially over the age of fifty, have much to gain from strength training by increasing bone mass and muscle strength. This is particularly important when you consider that up to *one third of all women who live to age ninety will break a hip*—a break that could be prevented if women take steps to keep bones strong.

The essence of keeping bones strong is *use 'em or lose 'em!* In our clinic, we believe that exercise may be as important as any new medicine in the treatment of osteoporosis. Each day we see the direct benefits of exercise, hence we take time to teach patients about the important relationship between an active lifestyle and a life free of this disease. Those patients who exercise more are the same ones who are more likely to improve. Likewise, those who cannot exercise have a much lower chance of improvement.

DIRECT BENEFITS

Stop telling yourself, "I am too old to exercise!" Everyone can exercise in some form, and age is not a limiting factor. We have hundreds of patients in their seventies, eighties, and even nineties who exercise regularly—not once or twice a week, but every day without fail. These patients say when they exercise they feel better. When they skip their daily workout, they experience more difficulty moving around that day. Some say their appetites are less on the nonexercise day, and mood swings and depressions are more apparent.

The benefits our older, active patients experience are very *direct*. For example, walking and other weight-bearing exercises strengthen the bones, which delays or actually reverses the process of osteoporosis. Exercise stimulates the cells that make new bone. By increasing daily activity, we encourage our bodies to form more bone.

The benefits of specific and intentional exercises are also direct. Take, for example, back strengthening exercises. As you strengthen these muscles, the bone density in the spine increases, thereby strengthening the entire skeleton.

INDIRECT BENEFITS

In older adults, the indirect benefit of weight-bearing and back exercise is improved stability and confidence that help prevent falls. Research has shown that weakness of the muscles of the back and legs is a major contributor to falls. When you add to the problem of weak muscles other factors such as less activity and diminished vision, you can understand why falls are a greater risk as we age.

Frequent falls can result in fractures and worse. Research has shown that with exercise and stronger muscles, a person's ability to stand and walk improves. Again, exercise can be as vital in preventing falls as new treatments are in strengthening bones.

HOW MUCH IS ENOUGH?

Scientists have yet to define the exact amount of weight-bearing exercise and back exercises necessary to improve osteoporosis. We suggest an optimal program of thirty to forty minutes of weight-bearing exercise at least three to four times a week, or more if you are able. Weight-bearing exercises include anything that puts pressure or resistance on bone—walking, biking, running, jumping rope, or climbing stairs. These exercises can be done out-of-doors or indoors with the help of a treadmill, an exercise bicycle, or a stair machine. (Note: Owning expensive exercise equipment is a luxury. You do not need any of it to protect yourself from loss of bone—all you need is a commitment to stick to a regular program.)

If you find that you cannot make a commitment of thirty to forty minutes, then break up your exercise into "mini workouts." These could be ten-minute bursts of exercise, such as walking around the neighborhood before work, taking the stairs at your office, parking in the back of the lot when grocery shopping, then riding a stationary bicycle while watching the evening news.

THREE TYPES OF EXERCISE

There are different categories of exercise that serve to build strong bones, including:

1. *Range-of-motion or stretching exercises.* These exercises involve moving joints as far as they will go (without pain) or through the full range of motion. The range-of-motion exercises will help you maintain flexibility, increase mobility, and reduce any pain you might feel from exercise or aging.
2. *Endurance and weight-bearing exercises.* When you

increase your endurance threshold with weight-bearing, cardiovascular forms of exercise such as walking, running, biking, rowing, or aerobics, you will not only improve conditioning but will also stimulate bone growth.

3. *Strengthening exercises*. These exercises help to build strong bones, muscles, ligaments, and tendons. Examples of strengthening exercises are isometrics and strength training using free weights, resistance machines, or resistance bands. Swimming helps to strengthen back muscles and increases flexibility without putting extra strain on the joints. It is an excellent form of exercise if you have pain and stiffness from arthritis.

GETTING STARTED

For most of us, starting an exercise program is more difficult than the actual program itself. Have you made a New Year's resolution to start exercising and found that the mere thought of a trip to the gym is exhausting?

Just as personal or career goals are important for success, so are goals for exercise. Planning exercise time is crucial, just as important as planning nutritious meals or getting regular, professional health care. Many patients say that morning commitments are the best for staying with an exercise routine. This keeps them from thinking of a myriad of excuses not to exercise throughout the day. Whatever time you choose, staying with it is important.

If you have been inactive for a long period of

time, start very slowly and allow ample time to let your body get used to the increased movement and activity. If you have had a recent fracture, start only when your doctor gives approval.

For those who have neglected exercise, a reasonable start would be to walk around your neighborhood block or take the stairs each morning at work. You may say, "Wait a minute. This is considered exercise? This is too easy!" Yes, it is easy. However, once you have accomplished this "easy" block or stair walk, I want you to increase the length to walking around several blocks or climbing the stairs many times throughout the day. You will be surprised how quickly the time and movement can build up.

If you have no pain or other difficulty walking this distance, increase the amount of time you exercise. Add five or ten minutes to the exercise until you build strength and endurance. Again, your goal is to be able to exercise a total of *thirty to forty minutes, at least three or four times each week*. Increasing exercise time slowly is better than overexercising and risking injury or burnout.

Once you make a commitment to your daily exercise program, stick with it. Use a calendar and check off the days that you exercise. Write down the time and distance you exercise each day. Your bones did not weaken overnight, and it will take months to build strength.

You will notice an improvement after a few weeks to two months, but whatever you do, *don't stop the exercises*. One patient diligently worked to build her bone mass with a daily walking program, increased calcium in her diet, and took medications. When she was told that her bone mass had increased by 3 percent, she stopped exercising! Once you realize your goal, keep exercising. This key step in the prevention and treatment plan must continue your entire lifetime, as long as you are physically able.

If you are unsure of how to start a program, consider seeking instruction from a physical therapist. A professional physical therapist can be sure you are doing the exercises correctly so that you get the maximum benefit. The therapist can also help you learn the proper use of moist heat, hot packs, and other helpful treatments, if you experience pain or stiffness during your regime.

BONE-BUILDING EXERCISES

AEROBICS (LOW-IMPACT)

Many osteoporosis patients have the idea that weight-bearing exercise means exercises that are high impact and high intensity. They complain that they are "too old and in no shape" to risk further injury with such activity. While putting additional weight on your bones to stimulate their growth is important to prevent osteoporosis, you don't have to injure yourself in doing so.

Low-impact aerobics are an excellent weight-bearing exercise, and many people enjoy exercising with others in a class. This type of aerobics also increases muscle strength with less chance of injury, as you put less stress on the musculoskeletal system than with high-impact aerobics. High-impact aerobics require much jumping around, and sometimes both feet are off the floor at the same time; low-impact aerobics always keeps one foot on the floor (i.e., there is less impact and less stress on your body).

BIKING

There are many benefits to riding a bicycle in preventing or treating osteoporosis. Biking is considered a weight-bearing exercise for the hips and legs, and it is an exercise that almost anyone can do, indoors or out. For those who prefer the privacy of their own homes, there are many types of stationary bikes that provide resistance, keep totals of distance cycled and calories burned, and are even low to the ground (recumbent bikes) for those who have difficulty climbing onto a standard bicycle seat.

Because the bike seat holds your torso weight, your lower joints do not receive the pounding effect that accompanies running or walking. If you are overweight or have joint problems in your knees, hips or ankles, biking may help loosen your joints while building supportive muscles.

DANCING

If walking or biking is not appealing, you might try dancing as a weight-bearing exercise to strengthen your bones. One report said that in a typical night of square dancing, the dancers covered more than five miles. An evening of ballroom dancing can be strenuous, weight-bearing, and an excellent endurance exercise.

ROWING

For those who have access to an indoor hydraulic cylinder rower, canoe, or rowing shell, rowing is a great aerobic exercise and can strengthen the neck, shoulders, and back, all bones affected by osteoporosis. Remember, a strong back is vital to skeleton strength. As with all exercise, be sure to check with your doctor before beginning a new regimen. Rowing can be especially straining on the heart and lungs.

RUNNING

If you are in good physical condition and suffer no joint problems, running can be an excellent way to strengthen bone and is a form of aerobic or conditioning exercise. If running causes you no unusual pain or stiffness, and you feel a strong need to run, do so with a few precautions:

- Wear good running shoes to give your feet and legs proper support.
- Run on soft surfaces such as grass on a playground or golf course.
- Take shorter strides to lower the impact of your weight on your joints.

If you feel persistent pain and stiffness after running, consider alternatives such as stair-climbing.

STAIR-CLIMBING

Studies have found that stair-climbing machines are as effective as running as an optimal form of aerobic conditioning and weight-bearing exercise. In fact, twelve minutes on a stair-climber equals a twenty-minute run. Stair-climbing allows you to have a full lower-body workout as you exercise muscles in your back, buttocks, and lower legs.

Yet if you have any knee problems or arthritis, avoid stair-climbing. Climbing stairs can put unneeded stress on knee injuries, causing joint trauma. The force put on the knees can be equal to several times the weight of the body. If you are not bothered with joint problems in the knees, hips, ankles, or spine and want to exercise vigorously, stair-climbing is a healthy alternative to running.

STRENGTH TRAINING

Strength training can be an anaerobic (without oxygen) exercise because of the constant start/stop motions. It helps to reduce the risk for osteoporosis as working muscles stimulates bone to help build strength. This type of exercise is also excellent for strengthening and building muscle, especially in the back.

No longer an exercise regimen for bodybuilders alone, resistance or strength training is becoming quite common for many elderly people, too. It involves using muscles repeatedly against a mobile, weighted resistance, such as you would do with Nautilus equipment or hand-held weights. A study conducted at the University of Colorado at Boulder looked at the effects of eleven men and women aged seventy to ninety-two. These elderly people—average age eighty—spent six months in an exercise program that involved strength training. Under close supervision they lifted weights considered heavy for their age and physical condition. By the end of the study all the participants showed considerable gains in balance and strength—some women more than doubled their strength in certain areas.

If your doctor permits, you can start a strength training program with careful supervision. Initially you should start using very light weights or resistance of only one to two pounds. At the beginning, concentrate more on form than the amount of weight you are able to lift. You can gradually add weight if proper form is maintained. Once you find a comfortable weight, you should stay with that weight for one to two sets of ten repetitions per body part, taking one to three minutes between sets to ensure a good quality workout.

WALKING

Walking is the perfect exercise and has broad appeal for everyone. It can be done any time and any place. This low-impact form of exercise is less likely to cause an injury than running or aerobics and provides the added benefit of cardiovascular fitness as well as strengthening bones and muscles and keeping joints lubricated and elastic. For those who do not want to walk out-of-doors, electronic treadmills and enclosed shopping malls allow you to continue weight-bearing exercise even in inclement weather.

A COMPLEMENTARY EXERCISE PROGRAM

Since almost everyone will have times when they are unable to get out-of-doors to exercise, we suggest a simple complementary exercise program that can be done at home. Researchers have found that the stronger the back muscles, the greater the bone density of the vertebrae. These exercises will allow you to strengthen specific bones in the body, as well as improve your posture.

Review the exercises on pages 99–103, and allocate at least ten to fifteen minutes in your daily schedule to do them. Keep in mind that it takes weeks to learn how to do these exercises effectively and to be able to complete the recommended number of repetitions. Yet with a strong commitment to the program, along with your thirty to forty minutes of weight-bearing exercises several times a week, you will begin to build stronger bones.

At first you may be able to do only one of the suggested exercises. It is important to note that in doing this, you should experience no more pain after you finish than when you began. If you experience severe pain as you perform these, stop. After a few days, try two repetitions of just one or two exercises. When you can comfortably do this number, increase the repetitions to three, four, or more, then gradually increase the number of exercises and repetitions. Your goal should be to work up to ten to twenty repetitions of each exercise daily.

As you are aware, there will be days when you feel good and see no reason to exercise. And you will have days when you feel bad and won't want to exercise. Do not go on what you feel! Remember, the more you stick with your prevention and treatment program, including regular exercises, the more certain you can be that osteoporosis and the resulting fractures will not affect you.

A physical therapist can teach these exercises and ensure you are performing them correctly. Ask your doctor for a referral.

BACK EXERCISES

Cheek-to-Cheek

This easy exercise can be done anywhere to strengthen the muscles of the buttocks that help support the back and the legs. Sit in a chair and press your buttocks (cheeks) together for a six-second count. Relax and repeat, increasing up to five, then ten, then twenty repetitions. Do this twice a day.

Tummy Tuck

The tummy tuck is an excellent exercise to strengthen your abdominal muscles, which, in turn, help support your back. You can do this lying in bed or on the floor, whichever is more comfortable. Lie flat, relax, and raise your arms above your head, keeping your knees bent. Tighten the muscles of your lower abdomen and your buttocks at the same time to flatten your back against the floor or bed. Hold for six seconds. Relax and repeat two or three times to start and work gradually to five, then ten, then twenty repetitions.

This exercise can also be done standing up or sitting in a chair but probably requires some dem-

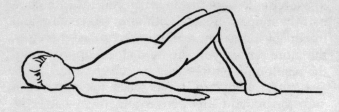

Figure 6.1 – Bottoms Up

onstration by a physical therapist for these positions.

Bottoms Up (Figure 6.1)

This exercise strengthens back muscles and is done lying in bed or on the floor (see figure 6.1). Feet are flat on the bed or floor, knees bent, as you bend (flex) your hips and knees, lifting your hips and buttocks off the floor (bottoms up!) four to six inches. Keep the small of your back flat against the floor and tighten the buttock and hip muscles to maintain this position. Hold for a count of six seconds. Relax, then lower hips and buttocks to the floor. Repeat this exercise, gradually increasing up to five, then ten, then twenty repetitions as tolerated, twice daily.

Tummy Toner

This vigorous exercise will help you to build abdominal strength, which in turn supports the back. Lie on your back with your knees bent and your arms relaxed by your side. Raise your head and shoulder blades about five inches. Hold that position for a six-second count and slowly return to the starting position. Repeat this one or two times, then gradually increase to five, then ten repetitions. As with all strengthening exercises, count out loud during the exercise. This will free you to breathe properly while holding the position. If you experience shortness of breath, stop and consult your doctor or physical therapist.

Back Builder

In this strengthening exercise, you will lie on your bed or floor in a prone (stomach down) position. Use a pillow under your stomach for comfort. Lie flat on your stomach with your body fully extended. Raise your head, arms, and legs off the floor, but do not bend your knees. Hold for several seconds while you count out loud. Relax and repeat two times, then gradually build to five, then ten repetitions, twice daily.

Cat Camel

This exercise can put pressure on sensitive knees, ankles, or hands, so perform this with caution. Get on hands and knees with hands directly under your shoulders. Taking a deep breath, arch your back upward as a frightened cat does, lowering your head; hold that position while you count to six out loud. Exhale and drop the arched back slowly, raising your head. Do this slowly one or two times, then increase up to five, then ten repetitions.

Spread Eagle

This exercise encourages the body extension positions and lets you have a much-needed body stretch. Stand spread-eagle facing a solid wall;

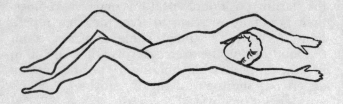

Figure 6.2 – Twister

arch your back inward slowly; repeat this exercise and gradually increase repetitions from one to five or more; repeat two times daily.

Twister (Figure 6.2)

Lie on your back with knees bent and feet flat on the floor. Raise your hands toward the ceiling, moving the arms and turning the head to the right, while your knees move to the left (see figure 6.2). Reverse and repeat. Gradually increase up to five, then ten repetitions daily.

The Bicycle

Lying on your back, move your feet and legs in the air as if you were riding a bicycle. Count to six, and relax. Repeat, then gradually increase to five, then ten repetitions once or twice daily, if tolerated.

CHEST AND POSTURE EXERCISES

Chest Expander (Figure 6.3)

This exercise improves the movement of the chest and helps your posture. On the floor, lie on

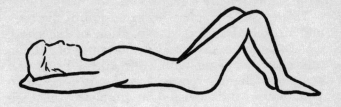

Figure 6.3 — Chest Expander

your back and place your hands comfortably behind your head, allowing your rib cage to fully expand. Bend your knees to protect your back (see figure 6.3). Breathe deeply, then raise your chest while filling your lungs completely. Hold for about two seconds, then exhale by drawing your upper abdomen in. In this position, take the next inhalation, filling your lungs completely. This may be a difficult exercise to understand without a demonstration. Contact your physical therapist or physician for assistance. Begin this exercise slowly, and gradually increase the repetitions from five to ten, then up to twenty.

In flight

This exercise encourages bending the arms and body backward, which helps to strengthen the back. Stand in a relaxed position, then lift your elbows to shoulder height with arms bent, elbows behind you, and hands pointed toward the floor. Straighten your arms backward and hold. Repeat this exercise and gradually increase the repetitions. Start with five and work up to ten, then twenty as tolerated. Repeat the exercise two times daily.

Arm Swing (Figure 6.4)

This exercise emphasizes extension of the back and neck and increased expansion of the chest. Good posture is extremely important when doing this exercise. Begin with your knees, back, and shoulders slightly relaxed (see figure 6.4). Begin with your hands crossed in front of you, then slowly swing them down and out over the head, reaching back as far as you can. When your arms are up, take a deep breath, and when you lower your arms, exhale. Repeat, gradually increasing to five, then ten repetitions, twice daily.

KNEE AND LEG EXERCISES

Knee Flex

Isometric exercises use muscle contractions without joint movement. This two-part exercise for flexibility and isometric strengthening can be done while you relax in a chair and watch television, on an airplane, or at work for a change of position and release of tension. These can be especially important for knee stability, strength, and standing support.

Sit in a chair and support your foot on a table or chair. Straighten your leg as much as possible and hold at that point. Flex your foot by pulling your toes toward you so the back of the leg is stretched. Then tighten your kneecap by pushing the knee down a little; hold the contraction for six seconds. Relax, and repeat. If this is done properly, you will notice wrinkles in the kneecap and the muscles in the thigh tighten. Begin gradually and work up to twelve repetitions at one time, two to three times a day.

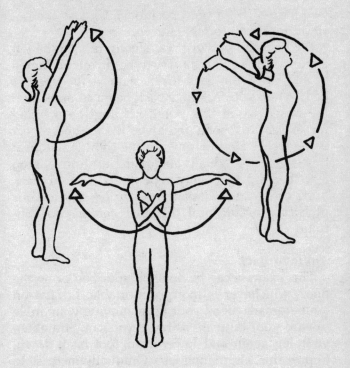

Figure 6.4 – Arm Swing

Leg Raise (Figure 6.5)

The leg raise helps to strengthen the large muscles in the front of the thigh (the quadriceps). These muscles are major support for the knee. This exercise also strengthens the muscles of the abdomen and improves the flexibility of the legs. To protect your back during this exercise you may hug one leg to your chest or simply bend the knee and hip, and rest the foot on the bed or the floor (see figure 6.5 for both positions). Choose the position most comfortable for you.

Lie flat on a bed or floor, slowly raising the left leg up as far as you can. Try to hold your abdomen in and press the back firmly against the floor or bed. When you feel your back begin to arch, stop the raised leg at that point, holding the position for six seconds; bend and lower the leg and repeat the exercise. Do the same for the right leg. Repeat this exercise, gradually increasing up to five, then ten, then up to twenty repetitions. If your back hurts or if you have pain in your leg, talk to your physician or physical therapist before you continue.

Ankle to Back

This exercise can be done on your bed or on the floor, whichever is more comfortable. Lie flat on your stomach. Bend your knee, moving your ankle toward your buttocks as far as you can. Straighten your leg again and lower your foot back down. Repeat this, alternating legs. Gradually increase to five, then ten, then twenty repetitions, twice each day.

SHOULDER EXERCISES

Touching Elbows

You may sit, stand, or lie down to do this exercise. Clasp your hands behind your neck and pull your elbows together until they are as close as possible in front of your chin. Separate the elbows to the side as much as possible. Repeat this motion, gradually increasing to five, then ten, then

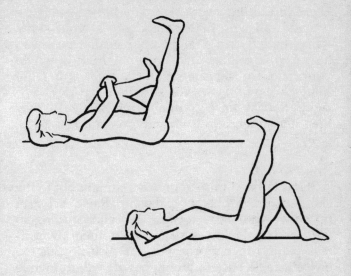

Figure 6.5 – Leg Raise

up to twenty repetitions. Repeat two to three times daily.

Hand to Back (Figure 6.6)
This exercise increases the flexibility of the shoulder and uses the same motions women use to fasten a bra in the back or men use to put a wallet in a back pocket. Stand tall and move your arms in the position shown in Figure 6.6. Continuing to stand, put one hand behind your back, then put the other hand behind your back, crossing the wrists as shown in the picture; return the hands to rest at your sides. Repeat this, gradually increasing to five, then ten, then up to twenty repetitions, twice daily.

Hand to Ceiling

Stand tall with both arms down at your sides. Raise the left arm straight up, reaching overhead toward the ceiling, then lower it back down to your side. Do the same with the right arm. Continue this motion as you alternate left-right-left-right. Repeat this, gradually increasing to five, then ten, then up to twenty repetitions, twice daily.

Arms to Side

Stand tall and raise your arms straight out to the sides at shoulder height, palms up. Raise each arm up above your head toward the ceiling, doing so with your palm up or palm down, then lower. If it is painful to perform, you can also do this exercise using a stick (a broom handle will do) while lying on your back. Holding the stick with both hands, raise your arms in front of you above your head as far as possible. The strength of your stronger arm will help move the painful arm more easily. Repeat the exercise gradually, increasing to five, then ten, then twenty repetitions, two or three times a day.

Shoulder Roll

This exercise can be done in a sitting or standing position and is a great way to relieve neck and shoulder tension during the day. Roll your shoulders in a forward circle, first raising them toward the ears in a shrugging motion. Then roll your shoulders back and stick your chest out as in a military stance; now lower the shoulders and finally bring them forward. Reverse the process, rolling your shoulder girdle in a backward circle.

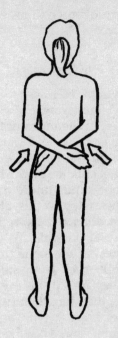

Figure 6.6 – Hand to Back

Repeat this exercise, gradually increasing to five, then ten, then twenty repetitions, two or three times a day, if possible.

Elbow Bend

Standing tall, raise your arm to the sides, bending it at the elbow and bringing the hand toward the top of the shoulder. Then straighten the arm completely, moving it straight out to the side of your body. Extend the arm fully from the body to gain full motion; repeat this five, then ten, then twenty times, two or three times each day. Repeat with opposite arm.

HIP EXERCISES

Knee to Chest (Figure 6.7)

This is a good limbering exercise to do before you get out of bed in the morning. It also stretches the hips, the lower back, and the knees. You can also do this one on the floor if you are able (see figure 6.7). Bend each knee toward your chest, one at a time. Put your hands under one knee to draw it closer to the chest. Repeat this, alternating knees. Do five, then ten, then twenty repetitions, two or three times a day, if possible. To finish, pull both knees to your chest at the same time and hold for six seconds; gently rock from side to side while holding your knees; repeat this exercise, increasing gradually to five, then ten, then twenty repetitions a day, if possible.

Thigh Lift (Figure 6.8)

This isometric, strengthening exercise can be done on the bed or floor, using a pillow under your stomach for comfort. You may experience some cramping when you do this because your muscles are working hard to accomplish this motion. If so, try massaging the muscle. If the pain or cramping persists, talk to your physician or physical therapist. Lie on your stomach with your leg extended. Raise one leg from the thigh straight up, lifting it several inches off the floor (see figure 6.8). If you lift too far, you will rotate your pelvis and will not get the desired movement. Lower the leg and alternate this exercise on the other side. When

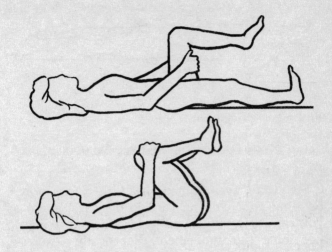

Figure 6.7 – Knee to Chest

you lift your thigh slightly off the floor, count six seconds while you hold the motion. Repeat this motion and gradually increase up to five, then ten repetitions, twice daily.

Knee and Toe Touch

This exercise can be done while lying on the floor or bed. It may seem like a foot exercise, but it actually rotates your hips when you concentrate on keeping your legs straight. Lie flat on your back; turn your knees in and touch your toes together; now turn your knees out. Repeat this exercise, gradually increasing up to five, then ten, then twenty repetitions each session; repeat this exercise twice daily.

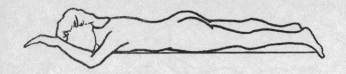

Figure 6.8 – Thigh Lift

NECK RANGE-OF-MOTION EXERCISES

Chin to Chest

Stand tall, eyes trained ahead, then look down, bending your chin forward to the chest as far as you can easily do. If you feel stiffness or pain, do not force this movement. Repeat this exercise, gradually increasing up to five, then ten, then twenty repetitions, twice daily.

Head Extension

Stand tall, eyes trained ahead, then look up, bending your head back as far as possible without forcing the movement. If you feel pain or dizziness, stop until you talk to your doctor or physical therapist. Repeat this exercise, gradually increasing up to five, then ten, then twenty repetitions, twice daily.

Head Tilt

Stand tall, head erect, and then tilt your head so that your left ear moves toward your left shoulder. (Do not raise your left shoulder.) If you feel pain or resistance, do not force the motion. Now tilt your head to the other side, right ear to the right shoulder. Repeat this exercise, gradually increasing up to five, then ten, then twenty repetitions, twice daily.

Head Rotation
Standing tall, turn your head left as if to look over your left shoulder. Try to point your chin directly over your shoulder. Go as far as is comfortable, but do not force the movement. Now turn and look over your right shoulder. Repeat this exercise, gradually increasing up to five, then ten, then twenty repetitions, twice daily.

MOVING MORE

Take advantage of the myriad of exercise opportunities as you begin an active program to build stronger bones and stay fracture-free. There are enough options to allow you to find the most effective exercise that you enjoy doing and that you will continue to do for a lifetime. Be sure to follow your doctor's instructions, along with the safety suggestions in this chapter.

SEVEN

The Wonder of Calcium

Calcium is important for preventing and treating osteoporosis. It makes sense given that calcium is the most abundant mineral in the human body. Women have about one pound fourteen ounces of calcium in the body, and men have just over two pounds. Of this amount, about 99 percent is found in the teeth and bones, the rest in other tissues and the circulation. While we ingest calcium daily through food sources or supplements, we also excrete a certain amount in the urine and feces. How do we replace the lost calcium? By making sure our diets contain enough calcium-rich foods.

The calcium recommendation for adults is approximately 1,200 milligrams per day (higher for teenage girls, pregnant and lactating women, postmenopausal women who are not taking estrogen, and men and women over age fifty). However, the average adult gets only two thirds to three quarters of that amount. In fact, some studies reveal that *80 percent of American women* do not get adequate amounts of this important mineral. Factors such as extreme weight loss can cause bone density to plummet to very low levels, and in some cases, it never recovers. Low calcium intake during adolescence can also limit peak bone density, as can certain medications and a host of risk factors.

Aging plays an important role in the efficiency of calcium absorption (see tables 7.1 and 7.2). Over our life spans, our bodies' ability to absorb calcium decreases the older we get. This is why a diet high in dairy products or other calcium-rich foods is necessary over the course of your entire life. For those who cannot get enough calcium through the foods they eat, calcium supplements and calcium-enriched foods are necessary alternatives.

A recent study on men and women over sixty-five had fewer fractures when they took calcium and vitamin D supplements.

Table 7.1
Age and Calcium Absorption

AGE	PERCENT OF ABSORBED
Infancy	50 to 70 percent
Childhood	50 to 70 percent
Adulthood	30 to 50 percent

TOO MUCH CALCIUM?

There are some dangers if you take excessive amounts of calcium, including the possibility of kidney stones. It does not usually help osteoporosis to increase your calcium intake *over* the recommended levels. Check with your doctor before you take higher-than-recommended doses or if you have had kidney stones or other medical problems.

Table 7.2
Some Factors That Affect Calcium Absorption

INCREASED ABSORPTION	DECREASED ABSORPTION
Vitamins A, C, D	Aging, menopause
Certain minerals and trace elements	Foods high in oxalic acid
Protein intake	Too much protein
Low-fat diet	High-fat diet
Lactose	Fast-moving intestinal tract
Gastric hydrochloric acid	Low stomach acid
Amino acids (lysine and glycine)	Stress
Exercise	Lack of exercise

HOW DO YOU MEASURE?

The Calcium Checkup (Table 7.3) is a questionnaire that will enable you to assess your past and present calcium intake. Try to identify any problem areas in your daily consumption of this mineral. Using this information, along with the host of suggestions in this chapter, you can do something to counteract osteoporosis, starting today.

START WITH DIETARY CALCIUM

If *yes* was your most frequently selected answer, use the information in this book as motivation for change. Learn the importance of a diet rich in calcium to build stronger bones or to maintain the bone strength you already have.

When the vast majority of people take the Calcium Checkup, then compare their daily intakes with the recommended amount of calcium in their diets as shown in Table 7.4, they wonder how they can consume what seems like a great deal of calcium. The fact is that it is not difficult to get your required calcium, plus the necessary nutrients needed to metabolize it properly. Read on!

As a rule of thumb, dietary calcium can reach the recommended amounts if you simply include three or four servings of calcium-rich foods each day. While calcium amounts vary in different foods, one serving is usually eight ounces of milk, one ounce of cheese, or an eight-ounce cup of yogurt. Milk, cheese, and yogurt are rich, readily available sources of calcium and have an added benefit in that they contain lactose, which enhances calcium absorption. If you are watching your weight, try low-fat or skim milk and by-products. They have just as much calcium as whole milk products, without the fat. Other sources of calcium include salmon with bones, sardines, and green leafy vegetables.

Table 7.3
Calcium Checkup

Answer *yes* or *no* to the following to see how your calcium habits measure up.

YES   **NO**

_____   _____   1. Are you allergic to dairy products? *(You may not be getting enough calcium from other foods.)*

_____   _____   2. Do you avoid adding milk or cheese to meals or casseroles? *(Dairy products, especially low-fat items, are an easy source of calcium to ensure strong bones.)*

_____   _____   3. Did you avoid drinking milk or eating dairy products as an adolescent? *(During childhood and teenage years, our bones reach their peak bone mass. Dairy products are a good source of calcium to help do this.)*

_____   _____   4. Do you take your daily calcium supplements all at one time? *(Calcium supplements are best absorbed when taken throughout the day.)*

_____   _____   5. Do you follow a strict weight-reduction diet that does not allow for extras like low-fat yogurt or skim milk? *(Strict diets frequently eliminate the necessary bone-building foods.)*

YES   NO

_____ _____ 6. Do you think that the recommended amount of calcium is just for pregnant women or elderly women who show signs of osteoporosis? (*A diet adequate in calcium is important for all people— regardless of age or sex.*)

_____ _____ 7. Do you drink more than two cups of caffeinated coffee a day? (*Caffeine may rob bones of calcium.*)

_____ _____ 8. Do you have a diet high in protein? (*Studies have shown that high protein diets also rob bones of the calcium needed to stay strong.*)

_____ _____ 9. Do you drink more than two soft drinks a day? (*Caffeine and phosphorus may leach calcium from the body.*)

_____ _____ 10. Do you have two or more alcoholic drinks each day? (*Heavy drinkers are at higher risk for low bone density.*)

Some foods that contain calcium such as vegetables may also contain oxalate. This oxalate may decrease the body's absorption of the calcium in this food. In such cases, even though the food may contain calcium, it may not be as available to the body as the calcium in other foods. Knowledge of this fact can allow you to include other sources of calcium, as well. Foods high in oxalates include asparagus, beets, broccoli, and spinach.

SUPPLEMENT WITH CALCIUM-FORTIFIED JUICES

Many factors influence the absorption of calcium. Much of the bone-building research has focused on the calcium found in dairy products and other food sources, but what about people who cannot eat dairy products because of allergies or for other reasons? Fortified juices may solve your calcium dilemma. Studies reported in *The Journal of the American College of Nutrition* (June 1996) found that fortified apple and orange juices may be even better at providing calcium than milk. Generally, we can absorb about 25 to 30 percent of the calcium from milk. Because of the different sugars and acid contents in juices, women in these studies absorbed approximately 36 percent of the calcium in an equal amount of fortified orange juice and 42 percent of the calcium in the same amount of fortified apple juice.

PLAN AHEAD FOR CALCIUM-RICH MEALS

As mentioned, you can easily incorporate high calcium food choices each day, but you have to plan ahead. Be sure to write these foods on your weekly grocery list and have them on hand for meal preparation. The following are inexpensive and easy ways to boost the calcium in your daily diet:

Table 7.4
Suggested Calcium Intakes

INFANTS	AMOUNT MG/DAY
0–6 months	210
6–12 months	270

CHILDREN	
1–3 years	500
4–8 years	800
9–18 years	1,500

ADULTS	
19–50 years	1,200
51 and older	1,500

PREGNANT AND LACTATING WOMEN	
14–18 years	1,300
19–50 years	1,200

Breakfast

Calcium-enriched orange juice
Calcium-enriched apple juice
Calcium-enriched cereal and skim milk
One cup of low-fat or nonfat yogurt
Carnation Instant Breakfast with skim milk
Hot chocolate made with eight ounces milk
Cheese toast or cheese sandwich using calcium-enriched bread

Sliced toast made with calcium-enriched bread

Lunch
Romaine salad with shredded cheese on top
Cheese pizza
One cup of low-fat or nonfat fruit yogurt
Milk shake
Cheeseburger
Bagel with cheese
High-calcium cottage cheese with chopped vegetables
Taco with cheese

Dinner
Chicken Parmesan and noodles
Fresh vegetables topped with sprinkles of shredded cheese
Macaroni and cheese
Cheese sauces over pasta
Bean and cheese burrito
Stuffed shells (Romano and mozzarella cheese) with sauce
Spinach quiche
Creamed soups

Snacks
Sliced low-fat or nonfat cheese and crackers
Fruity Bone Builder (see page 129)
High-calcium cottage cheese
Calcium-enriched juices
Frozen yogurt pops
Ice milk

Dairy sherbet
Sardines, with bones, and crackers
Rice pudding

Fruity Bone Builder

To make a delicious, calcium-packed Fruity Bone Builder, try the following recipe. Each drink contains approximately 500 milligrams of calcium, one half of an adult's daily requirement, and is low in calories and fat. Add your own extras such as chopped exotic or tropical fruits, honey, wheat germ, nuts, flavored syrups, or assorted flavored extracts. Get an extra calcium KICK by adding ¼ cup of powdered skim milk.

½ cup skim milk
1 cup low-fat or no-fat plain yogurt (or fruited yogurt)
¾ cup strawberries (or bananas, blueberries, peaches, and pineapple)
2 ice cubes
Sugar or honey to sweeten, if needed

Blend ingredients together in a food processor or blender until creamy smooth. Drink and enjoy!

VEGANS AND CALCIUM

Lacto-ovo vegetarians are known to consume more dietary calcium than meat eaters. While the calcium needs of vegans are not fully understood, studies have found that vegans may actually need less calcium than their meat-eating contemporaries. This could be because of the negative effect animal protein has on calcium absorption in the body. If you are a vegetarian, it is still wise to get the recommended daily allowances for prevention of osteoporosis as indicated on page 127. Also choose such calcium-rich foods as tahini, legumes, calcium-fortified juices, soy nuts, calcium-fortified soymilk, and molasses.

HOPE IN A BOTTLE?

Many women's magazines present new and innovative recipes for high-calcium dishes each month. Yet the truth is that most people do not eat enough calcium-rich foods in the quantities recommended. Some people cannot incorporate dairy foods into their diets because they cannot digest these products, and they are *lactose intolerant*. Their bodies do not produce enough *lactase, the enzyme needed to digest milk sugars*. Many people recognize themselves as lactose-intolerant because they suffer from telltale gas and diarrhea after ingesting dairy products.

In lactose intolerance, nausea, bloating and intestinal cramps occur after taking milk or milk products. But this does not remove the need for calcium to avoid osteoporosis later in life. An easy way to make milk products easy to digest is a product called Lactaid, which can be added to milk or taken separately as a pill. It contains lactase, an enzyme which helps digest lactose so that

Top Ten Vegetables Loaded with Calcium

1. Artichokes
2. Broccoli
3. Brussels sprouts
4. Cabbage
5. Carrots
6. Celery
7. Lima beans
8. Snap beans
9. Spinach
10. Swiss chard

The following nondairy foods contain enough calcium to equal an eight-ounce cup of milk:

5.7 ounces of dry roasted almonds
4 cups of cauliflower
2½ cups of broccoli or white beans
2 cups of rutabaga
1 cup of Chinese cabbage or turnip greens
½ cup of calcium-set tofu

the bothersome symptoms don't prevent the use of calcium-rich milk and dairy products.

For many busy people, the ideal goal of drinking three cups of skim milk a day, along with eating one cup of yogurt, an ounce of cheese, and a host of fresh vegetables, is unrealistic. And for millions of dieters, dairy foods high in fat and cholesterol are the first items to be cut from the menu. Thus, in these cases and others, more calcium supplementation should be considered as a cheap insurance policy for strong bones. However, which do you choose? When do you take them? How effectively are they absorbed and utilized in your body?

You may be wondering, "Why can't I just pop a few antacid tablets in the morning with my coffee and get adequate calcium this way?" Studies have found that not only is the *type* of calcium important for maximum absorption and bone-building, but the *timing and the food you eat or drink* might be equally important.

For example, research has shown if you are a forty-year-old premenopausal woman who takes the suggested 1,200 milligrams of calcium each day, yet you take the entire dose at breakfast, not all of it will be absorbed efficiently in the body. Did you know that if your calcium carbonate tablets contain 500 milligrams of calcium carbonate, only 200 milligrams are absorbed by the body? If you took calcium lactate, a tablet that contains 650 milligrams will have about 84.5 milligrams of calcium available to your body.

This means that if you were taking two calcium carbonate antacids each morning, thinking you were getting a full day's requirement, you need to think again. *You would need to take six antacids each day to receive the suggested 1,200 milligrams.*

WHAT SHOULD I TAKE?

Are there any rules to follow when taking calcium supplementation? Calcium advertisements on television and in magazines can often confuse the consumer as each claims to be the best way to build strong bones. Grocery and drugstore shelves add to this confusion as they are filled with a myriad of calcium supplements, from calcium carbonate to calcium citrate to calcium phosphate. While calcium carbonate and oyster-shell calcium are the most common forms, you may see calcium phosphate labeled as natural or bonemeal calcium. As if the choice of supplements available weren't confusing enough, there is a wide range of prices attached to them. Prices can be low for generic brands or outrageous for a name brand of the same ingredient.

So which do you choose? In many studies, calcium citrate has been found to dissolve easier than carbonate or phosphate. Researchers agree that calcium citrate is about 60 percent more *bioavailable* in the body. This means your body can use more of what you ingest. While calcium carbonate and calcium phosphate must be taken with food, calcium citrate can be taken with or without food. It has the advantage of producing no gas or constipation but is more expensive than other types.

The following tips may help you use calcium supplements to your advantage:

Tip #1: Avoid taking more than 500 milligrams of calcium at once. Spacing calcium supplements throughout the day is important as high doses taken at one time are not absorbed as well as smaller doses taken several times a day. Some research suggests taking calcium supplements at bedtime may help prevent bone loss at night.

Tip #2: Calcium supplements are best absorbed from the intestine when taken along with food.

This can be with a meal or with a snack. Lactose, which is the natural sugar in milk, and protein in foods help increase the absorption.

Tip #3: Avoid taking calcium supplements with foods high in fiber. Because high-fiber foods, such as whole-grain cereals and bulk-forming laxatives, interfere with the absorption of calcium, avoid taking your supplements with these foods. That's not to say you should avoid eating high-fiber foods altogether. A diet high in fiber is necessary to prevent many diseases, including certain cancers.

Tip #4: Do not take calcium supplements with high-fat foods. While a low-fat or moderately fat diet will not affect the absorption of the supplement, a large amount of fat can tie up the calcium and block its release into the body.

Tip #5: Do not take supplements with iron. If you are also taking iron supplements, be sure to take your calcium supplement at a different time of day. The calcium can bind the iron and thus limit the amount of either that the body will receive.

START THE CALCIUM HABIT

While removing risk factors for osteoporosis is most important, increasing your dietary calcium, along with the special "booster" nutrients you will read about in Chapter 8, is an important positive step over which you have control. If you are a parent, educating your child about osteoporosis prevention is essential. Talk with her about her body's

Table 7.5
Common Calcium Supplements

NAME	TYPE OF CALCIUM/ DOSAGE	ACTUAL AMOUNT OF CALCIUM
Alkamints tablets	Calcium carbonate 850 mg/tablet	340 mg/tablet
Biocal calcium tablets	Calcium carbonate 625 mg/tablet	250 mg/tablet
Biocal calcium tablets	Calcium carbonate 1,250 mg/tablet	500 mg/tablet
Calcium carbonate, liquid	Calcium carbonate 1,250 mg/tsp	500 mg/tsp
Calcium carbonate tablets	Calcium carbonate 500 mg/tablet	200 mg/tablet
Calcium gluconate tablets	Calcium gluconate 500 mg/tablet	45 mg/tablet
Calcium lactate tablets	Calcium lactate 650 mg/tablet	84.5 mg/tablet
Cal-Sup tablets	Calcium carbonate 750 mg/tablet	300 mg/tablet
Caltrate 600 tablets	Calcium carbonate 1,500 mg/tablet	600 mg/tablet

NAME	TYPE OF CALCIUM/ DOSAGE	ACTUAL AMOUNT OF CALCIUM
Caltrate 600+ tablets	Calcium carbonate 1,500 mg/tablet	600 mg/tablet
Caltrate 600+ D tablets	Calcium carbonate 1,500 mg/tablet	600 mg/tablet
Digel tablets	Calcium carbonate 280 mg/tablet	112 mg/tablet
Os-Cal 500 tablets	Oyster shell 1,250 mg/tablet	500 mg/tablet
Posture tablets	Calcium phosphate 1,565 mg/tablet	600 mg/tablet
Titralac tablets	Calcium carbonate 420 mg/tablet	168 mg/tablet
Tums tablets	Calcium carbonate 500 mg/tablet	200 mg/tablet
Tums E-X tablets	Calcium carbonate 750 mg/tablet	300 mg/tablet
Tums Ultra tablets	Calcium carbonate 1,000 mg/tablet	400 mg/tablet

calcium needs, and be sure she is getting the calcium required (see page 127) to build maximum bone mass before adulthood. Starting the calcium habit early on will help protect her future as she builds the strongest bones during periods of growth.

Ten Nondairy Calcium-rich Foods

1. Dry-roasted almonds
2. Kale
3. Corn bread
4. Collard greens
5. Calcium-fortified juices, breads, and cereals
6. Baked beans
7. Broccoli
8. White beans
9. Dry-roasted soybean nuts
10. Dried figs

EIGHT

More Nutritional Bone Builders

Who doesn't want to live longer? To reduce our risk of heart disease, cancer, diabetes, and other illnesses, many of us take the latest longevity research to heart. We focus on such lifestyle changes as eating low-fat diets with plenty of fresh fruits, vegetables, and whole grain products. However, as a physician who treats many patients with osteoporosis each day, I can honestly say that living longer is more attractive if you can also *live stronger*.

While the idea of preventing osteoporosis through dietary measures may be futuristic, this chapter will introduce the latest studies about bone-strengthening nutrients and specific foods that can help in the fight against bone loss. Some foods, such as soy and tea, may actually keep you from getting fractures. Researchers have found that in Asia, those who drink tea regularly may suffer less from osteoporosis. Other foods contain such nutrients as vitamin D, along with a host of trace elements—all vital for calcium absorption and metabolism.

Minerals other than calcium play a vital role in maintaining healthy bones. Dark, leafy vegetables, such as kale and collard greens, are abundant in magnesium. Scientific studies show that the mineral magnesium helps calcium gain entry into bone tissues. Boron, a trace element found in vegetables, seeds, and legumes, also appears to play a role in the metabolism of calcium and bone development. Vitamin D, which is necessary for calcium absorption in the body, is found in milk, fatty fish, and enriched cereals. When you combine the essential nutrients in this chapter with a high-calcium diet, as well as use the host of other preventive and treatment measures, you will be well on your way to staying fracture-free.

LET THE SUN SHINE

As explained in Chapter 7, calcium is the key mineral for building bones and keeping them strong. Yet calcium cannot work alone. It must have special "helpers" for it to be absorbed efficiently into the body. One such helper is vitamin D. Although this vitamin is found in some foods, most of the vitamin D used for building strong bones comes from sunshine.

Taking a fifteen- to twenty-minute walk several times a week should keep your body well stocked with enough vitamin D to keep bones healthy. Some studies show that because vitamin D is fat-soluble, your body can store it. This means that casual exposure to sunlight in the summer months may provide your body with ample amounts of this vitamin for the winter months. However, those who work in offices year-round may not be getting enough vitamin D if their exposure is limited to the sunlight that they get through window-pane glass.

Vitamin D has similar actions to a hormone in the body as it helps activate calcium and phosphorus into the bloodstream. Not only are these two minerals necessary for strong bones, they are also important in keeping muscles and nerves healthy. When the body has an insufficient supply of vitamin D, the blood levels of calcium and phosphorus drop as well. Where does the body turn to get more of these much-needed minerals? You guessed it—your bones. Loss of the minerals calcium and phosphorus is directly related to osteoporosis and a host of other bone-weakening problems.

Although most children and young adults get enough sunlight throughout the day to keep this problem in check, newer studies are finding that many older adults are in a different situation. Researchers have found that aging reduces the capacity of the skin to use sunlight to produce vitamin D. Therefore, daily vitamin D supplements of 800 IU (international units) per day beyond age sixty-five are suggested. Some experts suggest that even those over fifty should take 800 IU of vitamin D year-round. Check with your doctor about your particular needs.

The recommended dietary allowance (RDA) for vitamin D is 400 units. Along with sunlight, you can also obtain this vitamin from food sources, such as herring, mackerel, salmon, tuna, fortified milk, and fortified cereals. If you are not getting adequate amounts, you should seriously consider taking vitamin D supplements. A standard multi-vitamin has 400 IU of vitamin D and can ensure that your intake is adequate. Ask your doctor or a certified nutritionist to evaluate your supplements, as those greater than 1,000 IU may actually be detrimental to bone health and mobilize calcium from the bones.

While I am not advocating sunbathing by any means, some sun each day may help keep you a safe distance away from osteoporosis.

Table 8.1
Factors That Hinder Vitamin D Absorption from the Skin

- Increase in skin pigmentation
- Aging
- Topical application of sunscreen
- Windowpane glass that blocks natural sunlight
- Latitude
- Season
- Time of day

MINERALS

Not only is vitamin D important for the metabolism of calcium, there are a host of minerals necessary for calcium's absorption in the body, including boron, copper, fluoride, magnesium, manganese, phosphorus, and zinc. Although the specific role these minerals play in osteoporosis has not been defined, they are essential for normal growth and development of bones and play a prominent role in bone metabolism and bone turnover. The best way to ensure the correct balance of nutrients in the body is through a variety of foods, as they may be dangerous if taken in larger amounts.

If you are eating a well-balanced, nutritious diet, there is probably no reason to suspect you have a mineral deficiency. However, it is important to understand these minerals' function in bone health, as well as to identify specific foods that contain these. Three of the key minerals include:

BORON

Boron, another mineral plentiful in fruits and vegetables, appears to play an active role in the metabolism of calcium and bone development. Although the findings are still controversial, research by the U.S. Department of Agriculture indicates that boron increases estrogen levels in the blood. As such, it helps to create a balance of hormones (especially in postmenopausal women) and may slow the loss of bone. Interestingly, some scientists believe that this mineral might enhance estrogen's effects in women who take estrogen replacement therapy (ERT), and it may help to retain calcium and magnesium.

While there is no established recommendation for boron intake, you can get this mineral in plentiful amounts through fresh fruits, vegetables, legumes (dried beans and peas), dried fruits, leafy greens, seeds, and nuts. Avoid taking megadoses in supplements as there can be side effects such as headaches.

MAGNESIUM

Magnesium appears to play a key role in many biochemical reactions that are important to bone strength and metabolism. It regulates active calcium transport and may help to prevent fractures. Scientists have found that many older women with osteoporosis are deficient in magnesium, regardless of whether they are low in calcium.

Approximately 60 percent of dietary magnesium is stored in bone, while muscles and other tissues use the rest. The recommended dosages of magnesium range from 280 milligrams for women to 350 milligrams for men, and this amount may help in prevention of osteoporosis. However, some researchers believe that supplementing with more than 500 milligrams of magnesium daily may interfere with the calcium being stored in bone.

Food sources include cereals, nuts, sunflower seeds, tofu, diary products, bananas, pineapples, plantains, raisins, artichokes, avocados, lima beans, spinach, okra, beet greens, oysters, halibut, mackerel, grouper, cod, and sole.

ZINC

A growing body of evidence links zinc both positively and negatively with osteoporosis and bone strength. On the one hand, preliminary research suggests that a diet low in zinc may slow bone growth during adolescence, which might result in a higher risk of developing osteoporosis in later life. In one insightful study, scientists fed ten monkeys a nutritionally balanced diet including fifty micrograms of zinc per gram of food, while they fed ten other female monkeys similar diets with only two micrograms of zinc per gram of food. Researchers then followed the monkeys' growth from the onset of puberty at eighteen months of age through the adolescent growth spurt and first menstruation (twenty-seven to thirty-three months).

The researchers reported in the *American Journal of Clinical Nutrition* that the zinc-deprived monkeys had slower skeletal growth and maturation, and less bone mass, than the other monkeys. These studies concluded that this could show a possible relationship between diets low in zinc during adolescence and osteoporosis in later years, because the increase in bone mass during a female's adolescent years can be directly related to her risk of developing osteoporosis during late adulthood.

Recommended daily requirement for zinc is twelve to fifteen milligrams daily, but before you begin to stockpile zinc supplements, a word of caution: High doses of zinc are toxic and may, in fact, suppress the immune function. In fact, in older women, *high levels of zinc suggest reduced bone density*. Study after study has revealed that high levels of zinc may be related to *bone loss* in postmenopausal women. Until findings are conclusive, check with your physician for what is safe in your situation.

Foods high in zinc include seafood, eggs, meats, whole grains, wheat germ, nuts, peanut butter, and seeds; tea and coffee may hinder absorption.

RECOMMENDED AMOUNTS

The recommended dietary allowances (RDA) are issued by the Food and Nutrition Board of the National Academy of Sciences. These suggested amounts are the levels of nutrients that are "adequate" to meet the known nutrient needs of most healthy persons. This means that the RDAs will help to prevent deficiency-related diseases, such as beriberi or scurvy. There is now overwhelming scientific evidence available that indicates certain nutrients are crucial for disease prevention. One study showed vitamin E may protect against heart disease when taken in greater amounts than the RDA. However, the RDAs have simply not kept up with the scientific breakthroughs.

So how do you know what is safe and what is not? This is easily addressed by choosing foods from the USDA's food guide pyramid (see Table 8.2). Choosing a variety of healthful foods from the suggested groups, focusing mainly on a variety of nutrient-dense fruits and vegetables, will ensure that you are getting the necessary amount of vitamins and minerals. Or you might choose to take a vitamin and mineral supplement to ensure the recommended dosage. Of course, as stated in Chapter 7, calcium supplementation is still mandated if you are not taking in enough high-calcium or dairy foods.

Test Your Supplements

To see if your calcium tablets or vitamin supplements are being absorbed, place a tablet in six ounces of vinegar at room temperature. Stir this every two to three minutes. Within a period of thirty minutes, the supplements should have disintegrated. If not, better switch brands!

SUPPLEMENT WITH SOY

There is yet another "wonder" food that may help in boosting bone strength and could even help save your life by preventing other diseases. Studies show that soy foods can reduce blood cholesterol levels and the risk of heart disease, along with providing protection against certain cancers. There is also some evidence eating a high-soy diet may be beneficial in fighting osteoporosis and keeping bones strong.

Soybeans are low in fat and high in essential amino acids and protein. They also contain no cholesterol or lactose. For years soybeans have played an integral part in the Asian culture, with some positive health benefits. In fact, breast cancer rates

Table 8.2

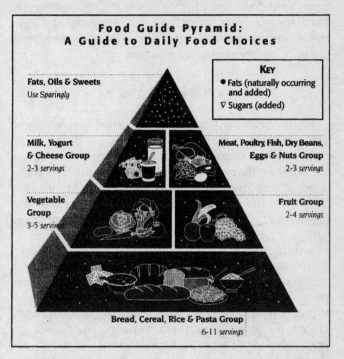

Food Guide Pyramid:
A Guide to Daily Food Choices

KEY
- Fats (naturally occurring and added)
- ▽ Sugars (added)

Fats, Oils & Sweets
Use Sparingly

Milk, Yogurt & Cheese Group
2-3 servings

Meat, Poultry, Fish, Dry Beans, Eggs & Nuts Group
2-3 servings

Vegetable Group
3-5 servings

Fruit Group
2-4 servings

Bread, Cereal, Rice & Pasta Group
6-11 servings

for Japanese women are four times lower than for those in the United States. Scientists believe the lower incidence in Japan is related to Japanese women's blood levels of phytoestrogen, which are ten to forty times higher than those of their Western peers. (Phytoestrogens are found in certain foods and mimic the work of the hormone estrogen in the body without the deleterious side effects.) Some of the latest research also points toward soy foods in relieving menopausal symptoms, such as hot flashes. In effect, it acts as a natural hormonal supplement. Soy's phytoestrogens may reduce circulating ovarian steroids and adrenal androgens and even lengthen the menstrual cycle of premenopausal women.

ISOFLAVONES ARE THE KEYS

In the body, the isoflavones found in soy foods are converted into phytoestrogens or plant compounds that mimic estrogen, although they are a lot weaker than human estrogen (about five hundred to one thousand times weaker). While the isoflavones may "look and act" like estrogen in the body, unlike human estrogen, they have not been linked by researchers to cancer.

Studies have found that like estrogen replacement therapy, high levels of this plant compound can also relieve vaginal dryness and other menopausal symptoms that frequently occur because of plummeting estrogen levels during menopause. Other hormone-dependent cancers may also be prevented by these plant estrogens, as well, although the research is too new to be conclusive.

Soy foods are the only source of *genistein*, a particular type of isoflavone that is a powerful antioxidant and appears to control unstable oxygen molecules before they change healthy cells into cancerous cells. Genistein blocks several of the key enzymes that tumor cells need to grow and thrive. For breast cancer, it blocks the receptors for estrogen on breast cells, thereby preventing estrogen from promoting tumor growth.

The National Cancer Institute is currently doing research on the potential of genistein as an anticancer drug. Not only is genistein being touted as a possible prevention for breast and prostate cancer, other cancers that are not estrogen dependent also respond to genistein. It appears to limit the enzymes that convert normal cells to cancer cells.

SOY AND BONE STRENGTH

While consumption of soy may be directly associated with a reduction of breast, prostate, and colon cancer in test populations, even newer studies show that adding one serving a day of soybeans may actually increase bone strength.

One recent study was conducted at the University of Illinois on sixty-six postmenopausal women who were not taking hormone replacement therapy. Of this group, the women who took in 90 milligrams of isoflavones (the phytoestrogen found in soy foods) a day for six months increased their bone density by *3 percent*, as well as the bone mineral content of the lumbar spine. The lumbar spine is the small of the back and is prone to fractures after menopause.

While the increase was small, it is important and offers tremendous hope to women who choose not to take estrogen replacement therapy at menopause.

In osteoporosis research, the isoflavones *genistein* and *daidzein*, two components of the soybean, have been shown to inhibit bone breakdown in animals because of their estrogenlike actions. Studies show that eating animal protein can weaken bones as it causes the body to remove calcium quicker. In a breakthrough study, researchers found that those who ate soy protein instead of animal protein lost

50 percent less calcium in the urine, thus helping to keep bones dense and strong. Because some Japanese women have half the rate of hip fractures as women in the United States, preliminary studies suggest that not only does soy help in blocking cancer and heart disease, soy may be the key factor in helping to retain bone mass.

QUEEN OF THE PLANT PROTEINS

Soy also has the highest-quality protein of any plant food, containing all eight essential acids. However, this ancient bean still appears to mystify most cooks. You may question the taste of soy food, thinking back to a time when you bought bean curd or tofu that was swimming around in a pool of murky white liquid.

Today's soy products are nothing like the white, mushy foods of the past. They come in many different forms and are generally very mild tasting. Not only does soy come in a myriad of forms, it can also be smoked or marinated and will take on the flavor of the dish it is used in, such as sauces, chili, dips, stir fries, fruit shakes, or pasta dishes.

The following soy products represent just a few that are available at supermarkets, natural food stores, and Asian markets:

Isolated soy protein. This is a powder form of soy protein that has a myriad of uses as you add it to casseroles, pasta dishes, drinks, and more. One ounce contains approximately twenty-three grams of soy protein.

Miso. This rich, salty paste made from soybeans and grains is aged for one to three years in wooden vats. Used to flavor soups, sauces, and marinades, miso can taste delicate and sweet to savory and salty. While miso contains isoflavones, since the serving size is small (one teaspoon), you only get a minimal amount of benefit.

Soya flour. This finely ground powder has more flavor than soy flour and is milder in taste. One half cup provides twenty grams of soy protein.

Soybeans. These dried soybeans have a delicious nutty flavor and can be used in recipes such as baked beans or chili. Just remember to soak them first as you would any dried bean. You can add them to soups or use them in any recipe that calls for lentils. One half cup provides 14.3 grams of soy protein.

Soy flour. Soy flour is made from roasted soybeans that are ground into a very fine powder. You can purchase this in defatted, low-fat, or full-fat versions. One half cup of full-fat soy flour contains 15 grams of soy protein, while the defatted soy flour has 24 grams of soy protein. Use soy flour to replace up to one fourth of regular flour in recipes.

Soy granules. These are tasty, nutlike granules that shake directly out of the container. You can soak these, then use them for a filler in recipes or sprinkle them directly on foods such as ice cream or yogurt. Soy granules have twenty-three grams of soy protein per one fourth cup.

Soy milk. This liquid can be used in virtually any recipe that calls for milk, and the added benefit is that eight ounces contains approximately ten grams of soy protein. Be sure and look for soy milk that is calcium-fortified.

Tempeh. This thin cake is made from fermented soybeans. It has an interesting nutty or smoky taste and chewy texture, and four ounces contain almost seventeen grams of soy protein. Tempeh is frequently used as a substitute for beef and contains more whole soybeans and fiber than soy milk or tofu.

Textured soy protein (TVP). This is a quick-cooking meat substitute made from low-fat soy flour that can be used as a beef substitute for burgers, chili, sloppy Joes, and more. It is available in many forms including strips, chunks, flakes, and granular. One half-cup serving has eleven grams of soy protein. Veggie burgers made with soy protein may or may not have isoflavones as some processed soy foods have had the isoflavones removed.

Tofu. This soy product is also called bean curd. It is a tasteless food, but by blending it with herbs, spices, and other foods, it becomes very appetizing. Tofu comes in a myriad of varieties, including soft, firm, extrafirm, and silken, and is available in regular and low-fat forms, too. Four ounces of firm tofu contain nine to thirteen grams of soy protein; the same amount of soft tofu contains nine grams of soy protein. Watch out for the fat in tofu. A three-ounce portion of "lite" tofu contains about one gram of fat while the same portion of regular firm tofu contains up to seven grams.

SIMPLE SOY SOLUTIONS

Researchers have concluded that eating approximately twenty-five grams of soy protein a day can assist in reducing heart disease. However, scientists are still not in agreement as to how much soy protein is needed for bone health. It is thought that the ideal goal is in the range of thirty to fifty mil-

Table 8.3
Foods High in Isoflavones

FOOD	SERVING	ISOFLAVONES (MG)	CALORIES	FAT (G)
Nutlettes*	1/2 cup	122	140	1.5
Roasted soy nuts	1/4 cup	62	195	9.5
Tempeh	1/2 cup	35	165	6
Low-fat tofu	1/2 cup	35	45–75	1.5–2.5
Regular tofu	1/2 cup	35	105–120	5.5–6.5
Soy milk	1 cup	30	120–150	4
Low-fat soy milk	1 cup	20	90–120	2

*Nutlettes is a crunchy breakfast cereal that can be ordered from Dixie USA, Inc., at (800) 347-3494. It provides twenty-five grams of soy protein per one half cup.

ligrams of isoflavones a day, which can vary depending on the soy product eaten. For example, the crunchy breakfast cereal Nutlettes provides 122 milligrams of isoflavones and twenty-five grams of soy protein. This isoflavone amount exceeds the ideal goal; however, those who live in Asia probably consume as much as one hundred milligrams of isoflavones a day, as do vegetarians who regularly eat tofu and other soy products.

You can start to incorporate isoflavones in your diet by replacing an animal protein with soy protein at one meal per day, then add more soy to enhance other meals and recipes. You're not sacrificing flavor by adding soy to your recipes; remember, soy actually absorbs the flavor of the food it is prepared with. Check your frozen food department for prepackaged soy products that taste like the real food item, such as sausage or ground meat.

The following represent just a few of the many easy and appetizing ways you can incorporate soy in your menu:

- Use silken tofu in desserts such as tofu shakes and puddings.
- Use tofu to replace ground beef. Crumble tofu and toss in spaghetti sauce, chili, tacos, or sloppy Joe sandwiches.
- Substitute tofu for cream cheese when making dips. Blend with chopped vegetables, spices, or prepackaged dip mixes.
- Use tofu as a topping for pizza or as a cheese substitute in pasta recipes.
- Use tofu as a dairy substitute in cream-based sauces and soups.
- Use miso to flavor soups, sauces, and marinades.
- Use miso instead of cream cheese in party dips for an added zip.
- Cut up miso and toss in a vegetarian stir fry to give more flavor.
- Use soy milk to replace cow's milk in the Fruity Bone Builders (page 129). A ratio of three-fourths cup yogurt to one-half cup soy milk makes for a creamy-textured drink.
- Use soy milk instead of cow's milk when making puddings, sauces, and pie fillings.
- Drink plain or flavored soy milks instead of cow's milk with meals.

- Pour soy milk over hot and cold cereals.
- Use in coffee or teas as a lightener instead of cream.
- Use soy granules to sprinkle from the container on cereal, yogurt, or ice cream.
- Add soy granules to meat loaf, stews, casseroles, and baked goods.
- Grill tempeh, coat with barbecue sauce, and serve on a bun.
- Use a quarter cup of isolated soy protein powder with every cup of ricotta cheese when making pasta dishes.
- Make egg salad using firm tofu as a replacement for chopped eggs.

NINE

Watching Out for the "Bone Robbers"

In our clinic we believe that prevention of any chronic disease should be approached in an "orderly" manner. This means if you first understand your risk factors and work on those over which you have control, you may greatly reduce your chance of having that particular disease. This approach definitely holds true with osteoporosis. Ending fractures starts with a thorough assessment of your personal risk, then stopping the destructive lifestyle habits that are detrimental to the health of your bones.

There are some specific "bone robbers" that can easily be controlled. We mentioned cigarette smoking and heavy alcohol drinking earlier in the book. However, there are other "bone robbers" you may not be unaware of. For example, a diet high in sodium and protein intake may cause increased urinary loss and negative calcium balance. Likewise, a diet high in caffeine intake also causes loss of bone calcium. Let's evaluate the top bone robbers, along with ways to control the problem.

NEW GROUNDS FOR DEBATE

Coffee and cola may be bone robbers to be concerned about. Breakthrough studies have revealed that excessive caffeine might contribute to osteoporosis. In one study performed on Harvard nurses, the risk of hip fracture among those who consumed the most caffeine (more than six cups of coffee a day) was almost three times higher than for those who did not consume caffeine. Other studies indicate that as few as two cups a day have been found to weaken bone and increase the risk of fractures.

As with all the bone robbers discussed in this book, there are steps you can take to counteract the caffeine/bone loss imbalance. We suggest adding more calcium supplementation to your diet or *drinking one cup of milk per cup of coffee* to help offset this negative calcium balance.

PROTEIN

It is ironic that in a nation where consumption of dairy foods ranks among the highest per capita in the world, American women suffer one of the world's highest rates of osteoporosis. While many variables are involved in the high incidence, one important factor may be a diet that is too high in protein, specifically animal protein such as meat and fish. Too much dairy—much more than the recommended amounts—may also be another key player in bone loss. While dairy products are high in calcium, they are also high in protein. In con-

Table 9.1
Bone-Robbing High-Caffeine Foods

Coffee, drip	5 oz	90–115 mg
Coffee, perk	5 oz	60–125 mg
Coffee, instant	5 oz	60–80 mg
Coffee, decaf	5 oz	2–5 mg
Tea, steeped 5 min.	5 oz	40–100 mg
Tea, steeped 3 min.	5 oz	20–50 mg
Hot cocoa	5 oz	30 mg
Cola soft drink	12 oz	45 mg
Chocolate bar	2 oz	30 mg

trast to the high incidence of osteoporosis and fractures in the United States, in countries where the intake of animal protein is low, there is also a lower incidence of hip fractures.

Protein is made up of amino acids. When these are digested in the body, they increase the acidity of the blood. Your body releases a substance that neutralizes acid in the blood in response to the increased acidity. The one acid-neutralizing substance that is usually available is calcium, which is stored in the bones.

Study after study has shown that as protein consumption increases, so does calcium excretion in the urine. When excess protein is digested, it binds to calcium and flushes the mineral out of your body. Even in young women, increasing dietary protein increases markers of bone turnover. Some revealing studies have suggested that many vegetarians have greater bone density than omnivores (plant and meat eaters) because of the reduced calcium excretion in their urine.

One way of reducing this effect of high protein on bone loss is to limit the amount of animal protein you eat each day. Check with your doctor or a certified nutritionist for the amount that is healthful for you. Another way is to replace animal protein with soy protein. Studies have shown that while isoflavones are being targeted as a crucial factor in preserving bone health (see page 148), protein found in soy, regardless of its isoflavone content, may also protect against the increased risk for fracture. Tofu, soy milk and soybeans are all high in soy protein and isoflavones and make healthy meat substitutes.

A SALTY SHAKEUP

It is no news that salt intake plays an important role in determining blood pressure. But did you know that it affects increased resorption of bone? Patients with essential hypertension are known to have increased urinary calcium excretion, and hypertension is another factor that may increase the likelihood of osteoporosis.

Nevertheless, some revealing new studies show that sodium restriction reduces calcium excretion and may reduce bone loss and hip fractures. One key study found that cutting your sodium intake by half allows you to retain about 18 percent more calcium. On the other hand, while some scientists believe that postmenopausal women who consume 3,000 milligrams of sodium a day need 1,700 milligrams of calcium (equivalent to six glasses of skim milk), others feel that this sodium/calcium connection starts much earlier, and that *women of all ages should be cautious about excessive sodium in their diets*.

How much salt is enough? According to a USDA survey, the average American consumes an average of 6,400 milligrams of sodium each day. That is the amount of salt in one tablespoon, but it is two and a half times the recommended daily maximum of 2,400 milligrams—remember, this is *maximum*.

Although the words *salt* and *sodium* are often used interchangeably, but they are *not* the same thing. Ordinary table salt is only 40 percent sodium. Too much sodium can increase fluid retention and elevate blood pressure in people who are sodium-sensitive.

Many foods naturally contain sodium, including animal products like meat, fish, poultry, milk, and eggs. Vegetable products are naturally low in sodium. Most of the sodium in our diets, however, comes from commercially processed foods such as cured meats like bacon and ham, luncheon meats, sausage, frozen breaded meats, fish and seafood, and canned meats and vegetables. Condiments like ketchup, mustard, and steak sauce are also high in sodium, as are fast foods.

It is a good idea to reduce the salt in your diet to prevent high blood pressure, fluid retention, and potential bone loss. Reading the ingredients listed on the package label to determine the sodium content will help you to stay within the

2,400-milligrams recommended limit. Using a variety of fresh and dried herbs instead of salt can enhance the flavor of prepared foods. Some favorite herbs include basil, chives, ginger, oregano, tarragon, mint, and rosemary.

Table 9.2
High Sodium Bone Robbers

Canned and dried soups
Canned vegetables
Canned meats (tuna, chicken, etc.)
Ketchup, mustard, and barbecue, steak, and
     soy sauces
Salty snack foods (potato chips, nuts, etc.)
Luncheon meats and packaged foods
Olives and pickles
Bacon, cured meats, ham
Fast foods (french fries, onion rings,
     hamburgers, Chinese foods)

STRONG BONES GO UP IN SMOKE

Although smoking appears to be on the decline in the United States, those who continue this habit are at a much greater risk of fractures. As discussed previously, cigarette smoking more than doubles your risk of getting osteoporosis. Tobacco may increase the rate at which you lose bone mass by reducing the effectiveness of the body's estrogen.

Smokers who are underweight are at even greater risk. The level of oxygen circulating in the bloodstream is often decreased in these patients because of such lung diseases as emphysema or chronic bronchitis. This lower level of oxygen may affect the way the body builds and removes bone. Also, the cortisonelike drugs that are used to treat respiratory problems increase the risk of osteoporosis and fractures because the activity of cells that produce bone is effectively decreased by those medications.

Even though smoking increases the risk of bone loss, not to mention the risk of developing respiratory problems and certain cancers, it is *one* important risk factor over which you have control. While you cannot control your age, your sex, or your family history of osteoporosis, you can stop smoking.

Sometimes it takes a serious disease to make one quit smoking, but you can have a head start if you make a commitment to stop today. You must recognize that cigarettes contain nicotine, a stimulant and addicting drug. When you stop smoking, you may experience irritability, nervousness, and headaches for one to two weeks, especially if you have been a heavy smoker.

It is important to remember that even for those who have stopped smoking for years, the urge to smoke can always return. It is a matter of mental self-control to stay away from cigarettes. Having the emotional support of an understanding spouse, family, friends, and co-workers is very important in tackling your addiction.

No matter how low your other risk factors are for osteoporosis, it is vital to your overall health and the health of your bones to stop smoking.

Soon after quitting, your ability to exercise will increase, which is another risk factor you can control. Even people who have smoked for years may notice an improvement in heart rate, blood pressure, and circulation to the hands, legs, and feet. If you have trouble stopping, talk to your doctor or call your local chapter of the American Lung Association or the American Cancer Society. Special aids such as medications, nicotine patches, and chewing gum are now available to help control the withdrawal symptoms when you decide to stop.

ANOTHER BONE-LEACHING HABIT

Excessive alcohol consumption is another bone-leaching risk factor that can lead to early fractures in women, as well as men. Osteoporosis is usually found earlier in life in those who have had a heavy alcohol intake for a number of years. Many sufferers who get the disease from excessive alcohol consumption are as young as age thirty to forty, younger than usual for fractures from osteoporosis. In fact, heavy drinking by women (more than two or three drinks a day) has also been linked to an increased risk of menstrual problems and early menopause, as well as osteoporosis.

Those who are affected with early osteoporosis from heavy alcohol consumption report feeling pain in the back, along with fractures, as with those who contract the disease from other causes. This is because alcohol's detrimental effect on bone tissue possibly results in reduced bone formation. Mineral and hormonal metabolism can also be impaired with alcohol consumption.

Often, people who drink alcohol in excessive amounts substitute the drinks for meals and become malnourished. This further intensifies alcohol's toxic effect on the bone as a diet high in alcohol is low in nutrients. For women, alcohol may have an even more destructive effect as there is less water in the female body. This means that the alcohol that is consumed is less diluted and can make a greater impact.

While alcohol consumption is an important risk factor for osteoporosis, it is one that can be remedied to some degree. If you drink alcohol, do so in moderation. If you don't drink, don't start now! Some recent studies have found that there may be a persistent high bone turnover after more than five years of alcohol withdrawal. This increase in bone is important to your strength in later years, so it is well worth stopping alcohol now. Keep your bones strong by eating plenty of high-calcium and nutritious foods, exercising, taking medications, if warranted, and getting fifteen to twenty minutes of sunlight each day.

WEIGHT LOSS AT MIDLIFE

While being at a normal weight is an optimal goal for most people, for some it could result in decreased bone density and increased risk of osteoporosis and fractures. A recent study by the National Institute on Aging has found that women who lose a lot of weight beginning at the age of fifty significantly increase their risk of hip fractures. The study focused on more than three thousand women who were sixty-seven years old and older. Researchers asked them to recall how much they weighed at the age of fifty, then charted their weight changes and incidence of hip fractures for eight years.

All the women in the study who lost 10 percent or more of their weight since age fifty increased their odds of fracturing a hip. This increase was greatest for the lean women—those who at age fifty had the lowest body mass as measured by their weight in relation to their height.

As stated in Chapter 2, women who are underweight have the greatest risk of hip fractures. The most obvious reason is that they have relatively low bone mass. They also have low levels of estrogen, a hormone that helps to maintain bone mass. And they have little fat to cushion their bones during falls.

But according to this study, it may also be that weight loss after menopause is a risk factor apart from low body mass. Researchers speculate that weight loss from a serious illness accounts for most of the increased risk of hip fractures. Perhaps this illness causes general weakness, which predisposes people to falls, and the weight loss causes bone loss, which increases the risk of fractures.

CAPTURE THE BONE ROBBERS

Some people may find it hard to believe that the "bone robbers" described in this chapter could cause osteoporosis over a period of years. Nevertheless, watching out for these specific foods and changing unhealthy habits are important ways you can continue to improve your goal of staying fracture-free your entire lifetime.

TEN

Staying Informed

Throughout this book I have encouraged you to understand osteoporosis—how it is diagnosed, the specific risk factors, and new measures for prevention and treatment that can build strong bones and end fractures. Open communication with a doctor who understands the latest diagnosis and treatment methods for osteoporosis is also important to gain a deeper understanding and to take control of this disease.

Read the following questions patients frequently ask. Then write down your particular questions and present these to your doctor at the next visit. The more you understand about how to prevent osteoporosis and stay fracture-free, the better your health will be.

Q: "I read about osteoporosis in many magazines, newspapers, and on the Internet. I know you say that it is possible to prevent bone fractures, but I don't know how to start. I am concerned because my mother recently broke her hip at age sixty-eight and is in a rehabilitation center at this time."

Sandra, age forty-four

A: The easiest way to start a prevention program is to check your own set of personal risk factors as outlined on page 34. If you have more than two or three risk factors, consider having a bone density test just to see where you stand as far as bone strength. The fact that you are a female, age forty-four, and your mother has had a broken hip, is probably reason enough to find out your bone density.

Depending on your bone density and other risk factors, you can determine your own personal risk for the disease. Many people prefer to guess about their bone health and worry about the disease, even waiting until they suffer a fracture to take treatment measures. There's no reason to do that.

The bone density test (page 41) is simple and safe. If your bone density is normal, be sure to follow all the steps for prevention as suggested in Chapter 4. If your doctor tells you your bone density is borderline normal, continue the prevention steps, then repeat the test in one year.

Most important, if your bone density is lower the next year even with a good prevention program, it is an excellent idea to add a bone-building medication, such as Fosamax. If your bone density is the same or higher, recheck the test in one to two years.

Once you know the facts, you don't have to spend all your time thinking about fractures and osteoporosis—just follow the easy steps to prevent fractures.

Q: "I thought osteoporosis was a woman's disease, but my sixty-five-year-old husband has become shorter and more stooped in the past few years. He took cortisone for five years for chronic obstructive pulmonary disease (COPD). At his age, does he need to worry about osteoporosis?"

Martha, age sixty-seven

A: Although more than 75 to 80 percent of patients with osteoporosis are women, men are also affected, but generally they show signs of the disease about ten to fifteen years later than in women. Just as with women, the first sign is usually a fracture, commonly in the spine, which can cause pain and lead to shortening and stooped posture. In some cases, spinal fractures happen without any severe pain.

Hip fracture is the most serious fracture from osteoporosis in men. It happens at an age that greatly increases the risk of death over the next year. After age seventy to seventy-five, hip fracture is one of the major dangers for a man's health.

Your husband's age, lung disease, cortisone treatment, and the stooped posture suggest that your husband might need to take steps to prevent future fractures. I suggest that he check with his doctor and consider a bone density test to allow proper prevention and treatment to begin.

Q: "I work full-time teaching school and rarely have time to exercise. You seem to emphasize exercise so much. Is this really so important?"

Teresa, age thirty-two

A: While exercise alone cannot prevent osteoporosis, it is a vital part of a prevention and treatment program. Research shows that otherwise healthy people lose bone strength if they don't exercise. Astronauts on weightless space flights, patients prescribed bed rest for a broken hip, and patients who must wear a cast on broken bones can lose bone strength over a few weeks or months. Evidence indicates that if back muscles are stronger, then bone density in the spine may increase. And it is scientifically proven that weight-bearing exercise can result in stronger bones.

Weight-bearing exercise and strengthening exercises are two great natural stimulations for bone formation. It would be unfortunate to miss the chance to use these treatments since they cost so little and work so well. But it may be hard to start and keep up these exercise programs unless you understand their importance.

Many of these exercises can be done at home safely and easily if you start slowly and gradually increase as outlined in Chapter 6. Walking or other weight-bearing exercise can also begin slowly and safely. Over a few months, you will be surprised how far you can walk and how many exercises you can accomplish without pain or stiffness.

In our clinic we find that those who succeed in keeping bones strong and preventing fractures are usually those who make a commitment to getting regular exercise.

Q: "My doctor recommended a bone density test because I have had several fractures. Now she thinks I may have osteoporosis. At seventy years old, I am concerned about exposing myself to X-ray radiation. Are these new tests safe or should I be concerned?"

Sarah, age seventy

A: These tests can be done very safely. If you are concerned about radiation, you may feel better knowing that the most widely used test, the DXA test (page 45), would expose you to extremely low levels of radiation. This is about as much as you might receive from cosmic radiation on an airline flight across the United States, and much less radiation than a routine chest X ray. Because these tests are not done frequently, they're very safe.

Instead of worrying about extremely low radiation, you should be more concerned about the danger of fractures. If you have had several fractures, your chances of having osteoporosis are high. Researchers have found that if you have a fracture after age forty, along with a T-score of -1 on your bone density test, your chance of hip fracture may be four or five times normal. A hip fracture at your age would limit your walking and independence, and carries an even higher risk of death, not counting the suffering and expense of the hospital stay.

Listen to your doctor. The benefits of finding out

whether you have osteoporosis would truly seem to be worth the test.

Q: "I am prematurely gray. In fact, my hair started to turn gray while I was in college. A friend recently told me that this increases my chances for osteoporosis. I am healthy and exercise daily. Should I be concerned?"

Liz, age thirty-one

A: Although there have been some reports of a higher incidence of osteoporosis in those with gray hair, this is not backed up by conclusive scientific evidence. Researchers have suggested that gray hair by itself does not increase the risk of bone loss. It is more likely that other risk factors were found along with the gray hair.

A good idea would be to look at your personal risk factors for the disease. Exercising daily is one important way to keep your bones strong, and you are at the perfect age to begin other prevention measures. If you do have more than two or three risk factors, then you should have a bone density test. Remove the risk factors over which you have control, and if gray hair is the major risk, then feel confident that it by itself cannot lead to osteoporosis.

Q: "I recently found out that I have osteoporosis after I fell and broke my wrist. My doctor told me to take extra calcium, but I had kidney stones a few years ago and was told to avoid calcium. What should I do?"

Becky, age forty-eight

A: It can be confusing when the treatments for two problems seem to conflict. First, see your doctor to be sure no other causes of osteoporosis are present. Then try to remove as many risk factors for osteoporosis as possible, and add an exercise program. Your doctor can tell whether you need to also include one of the medications to build bone strength.

In normal people, 1,500 milligrams total calcium intake per day does not usually raise the risk of kidney stones. In fact, that is what we recommend in our clinic. Higher amounts of calcium could definitely raise the possibility of stones. But everyone is different. The best idea is to talk with your doctor for advice in your own situation. There is a simple test called the *calcium urine test* which can measure the amount of calcium in the urine and help your doctor decide if your calcium supplement may cause more stones.

Q: "I am fifty-eight and recently tripped on a step getting off the subway, breaking my ankle in three places. After four months, I still have pain. Could osteoporosis be my problem?"

Lynnette, age fifty-eight

A: People who have osteoporosis do break bones more easily than those with normal bone density. It is possible that osteoporosis allowed the ankle to break with a minor trip on a step. It would be a good idea to have your doctor check your X ray to see if osteoporosis is present. And you should consider a bone density test, especially if you have any other risk factors.

Even though bones may break more easily, they should still heal with treatment. There may be other problems that have complicated your recovery from the broken ankle. Let your orthopedic surgeon guide you in this situation.

Q: "After my father died suddenly three years ago, I went into a severe depression that lasted for more than a year. I am now taking medication for this and seeing a therapist. I was feeling more hopeful about life until I read an article in a woman's magazine about a depression/osteoporosis connection. Am I now headed for bone loss and fractures at a younger age?"

Janet, age thirty-four

A: Depression alone probably doesn't cause osteoporosis. However, some researchers have now found that women who experienced a major depression had about a 6 percent lower bone density than other women of the same age who had no history of depression. There is scientific evidence that women with depression may remove bone more rapidly or build bone less rapidly, either of which could increase osteoporosis. The causes are not known, but higher levels of stress hormones in the body (cortisol) may be one key factor. Other possibilities might include loss of appetite with depression, which could lead to eating less nutritious foods, and decreased exercise and activity.

Until more test results come in on the depression/osteoporosis link, it is best to continue your treatment for depression and check your risk factors so you can keep your overall risk to a minimum.

Q: "My fifty-nine-year-old mother needed cortisone treatment for rheumatoid arthritis because the pain and stiffness were so severe that she was almost bedridden. She's better now, but doesn't cortisone treatment cause osteoporosis? What should she do?"

Rick, age twenty-five

A: You are right to be concerned about osteoporosis in your mother. The cortisone product generally used in treating rheumatoid arthritis is prednisone. Fortunately, low doses are often enough to control the pain and swelling in this type of arthritis. But the higher the dose and the longer the prednisone is used, the greater the risk is for osteoporosis.

Your mother is also at higher risk due to the fact she is female, postmenopausal, and has rheumatoid arthritis. If she has been inactive from the severe pain and stiffness, this would also be a factor increasing the possibility of osteoporosis.

It would be a good idea for your mother to talk to her doctor and check a bone density test. If she has osteoporosis, the earlier she starts treatment, the better chance she has of avoiding a hip fracture.

Q: "My doctor said I should start a medicine for osteoporosis to prevent fractures, but I can't take estrogen because I had breast cancer five years ago. What other choices do I have?"

Jill, age forty-nine

A: In addition to additional calcium and vitamin D supplements, weight-bearing and strengthening exercises, and removing other risk factors, three new medicines are available other than estrogen to help raise bone density and strength (see Chapter 5). This is important since it is known that if bone density increases, then the risk of fracture is lower, too.

Fosamax is a tablet taken once each day. Over 90 percent of patients on this medication show an increase in bone density. With this increase in bone density comes a reduced fracture risk. For example, the risk of hip fractures and spine fractures is decreased by about 50 percent.

As described on page 77, Fosamax should be taken thirty to sixty minutes before a meal, usually breakfast, with an eight-ounce glass of water. And you should not lie down before you eat. If you have indigestion, heartburn, or other new symptoms, then call your doctor before you continue the medication.

Evista (raloxifene) is a tablet taken daily. It is a choice for prevention of osteoporosis in those who would like to have the effects of estrogen in addition to the bone-building effect but cannot take estrogen. Evista can lower cholesterol without increasing the risk of cancer of the lining of the uterus or breast cancer.

Evista is mainly used for prevention of osteoporosis. Research shows it builds less bone than

Fosamax over one year, but does lower the total blood cholesterol and LDL-cholesterol (the bad cholesterol). Talk to your doctor to see if Evista is a good choice.

Miacalcin (nasal calcitonin) is a spray taken once each day to increase bone density.

Didronel (etidronate), a tablet taken for two weeks every three months, may also increase bone density.

Q: "My mother and grandmother both suffered from osteoporosis, and I have lost about two inches in height over the past few years. I certainly want to prevent fractures if I can, but I don't really know where to start."

Susan, age fifty-six

A: The best way to start is to learn about the risk factors for osteoporosis. If you have more than two or three risk factors, or if you have already lost height, it would be a good idea to check the possibility since effective treatment is available. Why wait for painful and debilitating fractures when you can take steps now? In fact, osteoporosis with fractures of the vertebral bodies is the most common cause of loss of height today.

Ask your doctor for advice. You should check your bone density test, which will tell whether your bone strength is normal or below normal. It can also give you an estimate for your own probability of fracture. Then you and your doctor can decide what steps should be taken to help prevent future fractures. Some newer medicines such as Fosamax have been shown to actually decrease the loss of height and decrease the rate of stooped posture.

If you need additional advice, you may want to have your doctor refer you to a rheumatologist, endocrinologist, or internal medicine specialist for further diagnosis and treatment of the osteoporosis.

Q: "I take inhaled cortisone medications for asthma and allergic rhinitis. Should I be concerned that these cortisone products might cause osteoporosis? I don't see how I could do without them."

Rob, age thirty-one

A: Although cortisone products such as prednisone and dexamethasone cause a higher chance of osteoporosis if taken over a period of time, the sprays used for asthma and rhinitis or sinusitis do not by themselves increase osteoporosis if used as directed. But don't forget that you still need to look at other risk factors, and remove those over which you have control to help prevent osteoporosis.

Q: "Are there any natural foods that could help build bone strength?"

Carmen, age thirty-eight

A: Research shows that there are some foods that may actually lower the risk of osteoporosis. This information has come largely from Asian countries, where there has traditionally been a higher intake of phytoestrogens through a diet high in soy. These compounds called isoflavones—found in many soybean products such as tofu, miso, and soy milk—may affect the body in several beneficial ways. They may lower the risk of osteoporosis, certain cancers, and heart disease.

Look through Chapters 6 and 7 and see which products you can add to your daily diet to help build bone strength. Taking all the precautions you can to stay fracture-free will be worth the effort, and using the many soy products available is an easy way to do this.

Q: "My doctor has suggested that I take a tai chi class. What is tai chi and why will this help me avoid fractures?"

Mary, age sixty-three

A: Tai chi is an ancient Chinese martial art whereby you follow a series of slow, graceful movements that mimic the movements you do in daily living. For example, you move forward, backward, and from side to side in a carefully coordinated manner—different body parts flow together as though performing one continuous movement. Followers of tai chi say that it speeds healing, improves circulation, boosts immune function, and decreases stress.

Some interesting studies have found that engaging in this Chinese discipline may reduce the risk of falling, and therefore reduce the risk of fracture. Researchers have suggested that tai chi helps to improve one's balance as the exercises focus on slow, continuous movement. Imagine standing on one foot without losing your balance. These movements and more are used in tai chi and give participants greater skill in counteracting any change in balance. For those who have experienced a fracture and have fear of falling, it may help reduce this anxiety and enable you to enjoy a higher quality of life.

There are books on tai chi, along with videos that you can use in the privacy of your home. Or contact your local YMCA or health club to see if classes are offered.

Q: "I had stomach surgery more than three years ago, and my doctor warned me about osteoporosis. How does this surgery affect the bones?"

Mike, age forty-seven

A: It depends on the exact type of surgery you had, but peptic ulcer disease and other conditions may require surgery to remove a portion of the stomach. In some cases, probably from the change in absorption of calcium and nutrients, people do develop a higher risk for osteoporosis. The best advice is to ask your doctor to explain specific ways to adjust your diet or food supplements to keep your risk at the lowest level.

Resources

Use the following resources as a guide to obtain more information on osteoporosis prevention and treatment.

Aids for Arthritis
3 Little Knoll Court
Medford, New Jersey 08055
(609) 654-6918

Arthritis Foundation
1314 Spring Street
Atlanta, Georgia 30309
(800) 283-7800

Arthritis Society
250 Floor Street East, Suite 901
Toronto, Ontario

CANADA M4W 3P2
(416) 967-1414

National Osteoporosis Foundation
1150 17th Street, NW, Suite 500
Washington, DC 20036-4603
(202) 223-2226

Support Group Services
National Osteoporosis Foundation Chicago Office
c/o AMA
515 North State Street
Chicago, Illinois 60610
(312) 464-5110
(312) 464-5863 (fax)

National Self-Help Clearinghouse (for referrals to
    support groups)
25 West 43rd Street
Room 620
New York, New York 10036

INTERNET SITES

Osteoporosis Links
*URL:http://raddi.uah.ualberta.ca/CAMOS/Other-
    Osteo.html*

Osteoporosis—Doctor's Guide to the Internet

URL:http://www.pslgroup.com/OSTEOPOROSIS.
  HTM

Osteoporosis: Not Just for Women Anymore

URL:http://www.texmed.org/comm/mediarel/radiospots/
  october/oct96ost6.htm

Osteoporosis (Diseases and Disorders)

URL:http://coyote.einet.net:8000/galaxy/Community/
  Health/Diseases-and-Disorders/Osteoporosis-1.html

Sympatico: HealthyWay: Health Links: Sites

URL:http://m2.medialinx.ca:1245/healthyway/LISTS/
  B2-C15-06_res1.html

National Osteoporosis Foundation

URL:http://www.nof.org/other/doctor.html
http://www.nof.org/other/calcium.html

Health Care Information Resources—Osteoporosis

URL:http://www-hsl.mcmaster.ca/tomflem/osteop.html

Osteoporosis

URL:http://www.emerald-empire.com/zines/health/
  menopa~1/osteo.htm

Health Quiz
*URL:http://www.statefarm.com/insuranc/health/hquiz2/
   hlthquiz.htm*

For osteoporosis information and studies
URL:http://www.tampamedicalgroup.com

Research and Supporting References

Arjmandi, B. H., et al. "Dietary Soybean Protein Prevents Bone Loss in an Ovariectomized Rat Model of Osteoporosis. " *Journal of Nutrition* 126(1): 161–67 (1996).

Binkley, N. C., Suttie, J. W. "Vitamin K Nutrition and Osteoporosis." *Journal of Nutrition* 125(7): 1,812–21 (1995).

Birge, S. J. "Osteoporosis and Hip Fracture." *Clinics in Geriatric Medicine* 1993; 9(1): 69–86.

Bonjour, J. P., et al. "Nutritional Aspects of Hip Fractures." *Bone* 1996 Mar; 18(3 Suppl): 139S–144S.

Bowman, M. A., Spangler, J. G. "Osteoporosis in Women." *Primary Care* 24(1): 27–36 (1997).

Chapuy, M. C., et al. "Vitamin D$_3$ and Calcium to Prevent Hip Fractures in Elderly Women." *New*

England Journal of Medicine 1992; 327(23): 1,637–42.

Chestnut, C. H. "Bone Mass and Exercise." *American Journal of Medicine* 1993; 95 (supp 5A): 34s–36s.

Dargent-Molina, P., et al. "Fall-related Factors and Risk of Hip Fracture: the EPIDOS Prospective Study. *Lancet*, 1996 July 20; 348(9021): 145–9.

Felson, D. T., et al. "The Effect of Postmenopausal Estrogen Therapy on Bone Density in Elderly Women." *New England Journal of Medicine* 1993; 329(16): 1,141–46.

Ilich, J. Z. "Primary Prevention of Osteoporosis: Pediatric Approach to Disease of the Elderly." *Woman's Health Issues* 1996 Jul-Aug;6(4): 194–203.

Jeal, W., Barradell, L. B., McTavish, D. "Alendronate: A Review of Its Pharmacological Properties and Therapeutic Efficacy in Postmenopausal Osteoporosis." *Drugs* 53(3): 415–34 (1997).

Johnston, C. C., Slemenda, C. W., Melton, L. J. "Clinical Use of Bone Densitometry." New England Journal of Medicine 1991; 324(16): 1,105–08.

Kanis, J. A. "Treatment of Symptomatic Osteoporosis with Fluoride." *American Journal of Medicine* 1993; 95 (supp 5A): 53S–61S.

Kelepouris, N., et al. "Severe Osteoporosis in Men." *Annuals of Internal Medicine* 123 (6): 452–60 (1995).

Kiel, D. P., et al. "The Effect of Smoking at Different Life Stages on Bone Mineral Density in Elderly Men and Women." *Osteoporosis Int* 6(3): 240–48 (1996).

Knight, D. C., Eden, J. A.. "A Review of the Clinical Effects of Phytoestrogens." *Obstetrics and Gynecology* 1996 May; 87(5 Pt 2): 897–904.

Langlois, J. A., Harris, T., Looker, A. C., Madans, J. "Weight Change Between Age 50 Years and Old Age Is Associated with Risk of Hip Fracture in White Women Aged 67 Years and Older." *Archives of Internal Medicine*, 1996 May 13; 156(9): 989–94.

Lieberman, U. A., et al. "Effect of Oral Alendronate on Bone Mineral Density and the Incidence of Fractures in Postmenopausal Osteoporosis. The Alendronate Phase III Osteoporosis Treatment Study Group." *New England Journal of Medicine* 1995; 333(22): 1437–43.

Lonzer, M. D., et al. "Effects of Heredity, Age, Weight, Puberty, Activity, and Calcium Intake on Bone Mineral Density in Children." *Clinical Pediatrics* 1996 Apr; 35(4): 185–9.

Margolis, A., Greenwood, S. "Menopausal Syndrome." In: Tierney L., McPhee S., Papadakis, M., Schroeder, S., eds. *Current Medical Diagnosis and Treatment*. Norwalk, Lange; 1994: 591–2.

Michaelson, D., et al. "Bone Mineral Density in Women with Depression." *New England Journal of Medicine* 1996; 335 (16), 1,176–81.

Optimal Calcium Intake. NIH Consensus Statement 1994 June 6–8; 12(4): 1–31.

Papapoulos, S. E. "The Role of Bisphosphonates in the Prevention and Treatment of Osteoporosis."

American Journal of Medicine 1993; 95(supp5A): 48S–52S.

Recker, Robert R. "The Use of Alendronate for Treatment of Osteoporosis." *The Osteoporosis Report, National Osteoporosis Foundation.* Winter 1995.

Reid, I. R., Ames, R. W., et al. "Effect of Calcium Supplementation on Bone Loss in Postmenopausal Women." *New England Journal of Medicine* 1993: 328(7): 460–64.

Riggs, L. R., Melton, L.R. "The Prevention and Treatment of Osteoporosis." *New England Journal of Medicine* 1992; 327(9): 620–27.

Rizzoli, R., Bonjour, J. P. "Hormones and Bones." *Lancet 349:* S120–S123 (1997).

Rubin, S. M., Cummings, S. R. "Results of Bone Densitometry Affect Women's Decisions about Taking Measures to Prevent Fractures." *Annals of Internal Medicine* 1992; 116(12): 990–95.

Sabatier, J. P., et al. "Bone Mineral Acquisition During Adolescence and Early Adulthood: A Study in 574 Healthy Females 10–24 Years of Age." *Osteoporosis Int* 1996; 6(2): 141–48.

Seeman, E. "Do Men Suffer with Osteoporosis?" *Aust Family Physician* 26(2): 135–43 (1997).

Swezey, R. L. "Exercise for Osteoporosis—Is Walking Enough? The Case for Site Specificity and Resistive Exercise." *Spine* 21(23): 2,809–13 (1996).

Taggart, H. M., Connor, S. E. "The Relation of Exercise Habits to Health Beliefs and Knowledge about Osteoporosis." *Journal of the American Col-*

lege of Heatlh 1995 Nov; 44(3): 127–30.

"Taking Hormones and Women's Health: Choices, Risks and Benefits." *National Women's Health Network*, 1995.

U.S. Congress, Office of Technology Assessment. "Public Information about Osteoporosis: What's Available, What's Needed?" Background Paper, OTA-BP-H131. Washington, D. C. Government Printing Office, July 1994.

Upritchard, J. E., Ball, M. J. "Fat and Calcium Intake in Women Dieters." *American Journal of Clinical Nutrition*, January 1996; 63(1): 67–71.

Index

191

HEALTH CARE BOOKS FOR THE INFORMED CONSUMER